My Guide Fibromyalgia/CFS

Rebecca Richmond

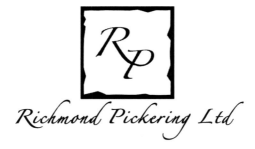

Richmond Pickering Ltd

First published in Great Britain 2013
by Richmond Pickering Ltd
Denmark Cottage
Lower Hengoed
Oswestry
Shropshire SY10 7EF

www.richmondpickering.com

British Library Cataloguing-in-Publication Data
A catalogue record for this book is available
from the British Library

ISBN-10: 0957237219
ISBN-13: 978-0-9572372-1-6

Printed in Great Britain by
Bell & Bain Ltd, Glasgow

Dedication

For my amazing and ever-supportive husband
and wonderful daughter.

Thank you both for your love and support –
which I hope I am able to repay one day.

Acknowledgements

There are far too many to list, but I am particularly grateful to so many people in the field of personal development and the understanding of the mind–body connection.

Also, Claire Pickering – my wonderful editor, business partner and friend.

Contents

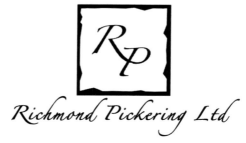

Richmond Pickering Ltd

Foreword

A journey of a thousand miles begins with a single step.

Confucius

When I developed fibromyalgia/CFS, my enjoyment of life gradually deteriorated – I realise many of you reading this book will know what that feels like and how it can devastate people's lives from personal experience. But what may surprise you is that I am now grateful that I developed it.

In discovering how to recover from my condition so that I can now live a full and active life again, I embarked on a journey using the immense power of the unconscious mind to enhance the way I think and behave, which improved every area of my life.

I have been able to use the skills and techniques I acquired to develop an amazingly rewarding career. Perhaps the greatest gift of all is that I firmly believe that developing a deep understanding of my body and mind saved my life.

It is my belief that the techniques I learnt aided my recovery from surgery to remove a pancreatic tumour. My ability to understand and consciously connect with my body was, in my opinion, directly responsible for the early diagnosis of my malignant melanoma.

☺ I gave a lot of consideration as to whether or not writing this book would have an effect on my health, because it meant reconnecting with my condition at the deepest level and re-examining all of my symptoms. The good news is it didn't and I am still fit and well.

My Guide: Manage Fibromyalgia/CFS is not an instruction manual. Neither is it intended to cure any illnesses or injuries you may have. It is simply my journey to recovery, in which I have explained the techniques I used to aid my recovery. This book is designed to share my understanding that fibromyalgia/CFS is not something that just happens. It is my belief that it is the body's way of telling you that you need to take action in some area of your life.

My life began to change when someone made me realise that the events in my life or, more importantly, my reaction to those events had impacted on my body. I will never forget what she said:

> You have really been through so much, rationalising everything and carrying on. Frankly, most people would have had a nervous breakdown. Even though you have coped, all that stress and those negative emotions have to have had an effect and it is your body's way of telling you it has had enough!

I am committed to helping people with fibromyalgia and chronic fatigue syndrome (CFS) gain emotional wellness and overcome their symptoms, taking one day at a time. My greatest wish is that you discover how to have a life filled with confidence, joy and vibrant good health like me.

This book is for people who understand or who are open to the idea that stress and other negative emotions can have an effect on our well-being. That doesn't mean that either condition is an imagined illness and therefore all in the mind – they are very real. But it is important to accept that there are ways you can reduce the intensity in which you feel pain.

Managing fibromyalgia/CFS is not about learning how to overcome the symptoms so you can carry on living your life in the same way you did before. It is about adopting a completely new attitude to life and developing an acceptance that life is going to be better in every way because you have found a new way to approach and enjoy each day. It is a way of being that leads to better health and emotional balance.

I was motivated to write this book as a result of the desperation and hopelessness of a group of sufferers and their families who firmly believed that there was no hope of them recovering. They felt that anyone who claimed to have recovered had either never been ill in the first place or worse, was a charlatan who was intending to prey on their vulnerability. Even if you believe that you will never recover from fibromyalgia/CFS, you can still learn how to manage and reduce the symptoms, and live a full and happy life. I sincerely hope that this book will inspire you to make changes in your own thinking so you can begin your own journey to recovery.

I had the pleasure of meeting an amazing lady who leads a group of sufferers in their search for a cure. She told me that I am one of only a handful of sufferers in the world who has developed their own system to recover from fibromyalgia – it is this system I will share with you in this book.

I will still be writing this book when I am ninety if I try to explain everything I have learnt about the power of the mind on my journey to recovery, so I have put together simple techniques that I used to help me recover that you can do at home. If you wish to learn more about my coaching methods and products, please visit my website at: <http://www.forgetfibromyalgia.com>.

Legal Disclaimer

Chapter One – Overview of Fibromyalgia and CFS

To get through the hardest journey we need
take only one step at a time, but we must
keep on stepping.

Chinese Proverb

Definition of Fibromyalgia

Fibromyalgia, also called fibromyalgia syndrome, is a chronic, long-term condition that causes all-over pain of the body and it is a syndrome rather than a disease.

The name fibromyalgia comes from the Latin term:

- 'fibro', meaning fibrous tissues – such as the tendons (bands of tissue that connect muscles to bones) and ligaments (bands of tissue connecting bones to bones)

and the Greek names:

- 'my', meaning muscles, and
- 'algia', meaning pain.

Fibromyalgia is referred to as a 'syndrome' because it is a collection of symptoms, rather than a disease. It is an illness that involves both the mind and the body. It is not arthritis because it does not affect the joints.

Fibromyalgia used to be known as fibrositis, which literally means inflammation (swelling) of the muscles and soft, fibrous connective tissue, causing stiffness and pain. However, after studies found that in fact there is no actual inflammation, the condition was renamed fibromyalgia.

About Fibromyalgia

Fibromyalgia is a chronic rheumatic condition that is characterised by muscular or musculoskeletal pains with stiffness and localised tenderness at specific points on the body. It is recognised that people with certain rheumatic diseases are more likely to have fibromyalgia. The pain tends to be felt as widespread aching or burning, often described as being all over the body, with even gentle touch causing pain that can last for days. There may be flare-ups where it is worse at some times than others and it may also change location, often becoming more severe in parts of the body such as the legs, neck and arms.

The fatigue ranges from acute tiredness to the exhaustion of a flu-like illness. It may come and go and people can suddenly feel totally overwhelmed by exhaustion within minutes, where they are drained of all energy – as if someone has just 'switched off the power'.

There is a wide variation in the level of pain and fatigue experienced by sufferers. While there is no reason to believe that all sufferers will deteriorate, most people find that at some time or other they are prevented from doing normal activities such as walking up stairs, shopping or housework.

Symptoms can be aggravated by completely unrelated illnesses, including hormone changes in women occurring especially around the menstrual cycle, changes in the weather and stress. Symptoms can be similar to those of CFS or myalgic encephalomyelitis (ME). Some people believe the two conditions are the same, but in actual fact symptoms vary and fibromyalgia sufferers can experience strongly disabling chronic pain.

It is estimated that fibromyalgia may affect up to 4.5 per cent of the population across the globe. Anyone can develop fibromyalgia, but approximately 70 to 90 per cent of sufferers are women. In most cases fibromyalgia occurs between the ages of 30 and 60, usually developing between the ages of 25 and 55. It is not common in young adults and children are rarely affected, but it can develop in people of any age.

What Causes Fibromyalgia?

The cause of fibromyalgia is unknown. However, researchers have several theories about causes or triggers of the disorder, some of which include:

1. An injury or repetitive injuries that have affected the central nervous system.

2. Genetic predisposition – although research remains inconclusive at the time of writing this text, genetic factors also may play a role in the development of fibromyalgia.

3. A physically or emotionally stressful or traumatic event such as a divorce, an accident or a death in the family.

4. Depression or a sustained period of stress. It has been suggested that fibromyalgia may result from stress-induced changes to the function and integrity of areas of the brain that control basic emotions such as fear, pleasure and anger, and the ability to judge distances.

5. Another illness or infectious agent such as a virus in susceptible people.

The cause maybe unknown and perhaps occurs for no reason, but the pain and suffering are very real and can cause a great deal of distress to both sufferers and their families.

Common Symptoms of Fibromyalgia

It is thought that people with fibromyalgia are unable to obtain the deep, restorative sleep their bodies need. This leads to a cycle of fatigue and pain. Someone suffering from the condition usually experiences aches all over the body, although there will be certain areas where pain is more localised. Some of the main symptoms include:

- pain
- fatigue
- sleep disturbance and waking up feeling exhausted
- morning stiffness
- headaches
- concentration problems – 'fibro (brain) fog'
- irritable bowel syndrome
- painful menstrual periods
- restless legs syndrome, where legs are uncomfortable and twitchy, especially at night
- poor circulation, with tingling or swelling of the hands and feet
- an urgent need to urinate.

Feeling tired a lot of the time can make it hard to carry out simple, everyday tasks such as housework or going to work. This can lead to frustration and depression.

Fibromyalgia is an invisible illness. This can mean people do not understand how bad you are feeling – which can make you feel even more despondent, discouraged and exasperated.

Fibromyalgia Diagnosis

Fibromyalgia is difficult to diagnose because the symptoms are similar to those of other illnesses and therefore it can take a considerable amount of time before an accurate diagnosis may be given, usually following a process of elimination.

No standard medical test or X-ray can provide a definitive diagnosis of fibromyalgia. People with fibromyalgia have tender points in certain parts of the body, which a doctor will assess to try to make a diagnosis based on the symptoms. Often, the medical profession will use the American College of Rheumatology's 1990 criteria for classifying fibromyalgia. According to these criteria, a person is considered to have fibromyalgia if he/she experiences widespread pain (occurring on the left and right side of the body) for at least three months, in combination with tenderness in at least eleven of eighteen specific tender-point sites.

Definition of Chronic Fatigue Syndrome (CFS)

The term chronic fatigue syndrome (CFS) is commonly used to describe a debilitating medical condition. It is generally defined by extreme and persistent fatigue, lasting six months or more and often accompanied by other specific symptoms:

- chronic – referring to an illness lasting a long time or frequently reoccurring

- fatigue – extreme tiredness, typically resulting from mental or physical exertion, or illness

- syndrome – a group of symptoms that consistently occur together.

About CFS

Chronic fatigue syndrome has also been called post-viral fatigue syndrome, myalgic encephalomyelitis (ME) or chronic fatigue. It can affect people of any age. However, it is most common between the ages of 24 and 45. It is estimated that about 150,000 people in the UK and approximately 1 million in the USA have CFS, with women affected more than men. It is also believed that as few as 20 per cent of the cases are reported. Children can also be affected, most commonly between the ages of 13 and 15.

- CFS stands for chronic fatigue syndrome. Chronic means persistent or long-term.

- ME stands for myalgic encephalomyelitis. Myalgic means muscle aches or pains. Encephalomyelitis means inflammation of the brain and spinal cord.

CFS is a condition that causes long-term, disabling tiredness (fatigue) that is not caused by any other known medical condition. It is often accompanied by other symptoms, such as muscular and joint pain, lack of concentration, headaches and disturbed sleep patterns. Treatments including graded exercise therapy or cognitive behavioural therapy may help in some cases, but there is no recognised cure.

Some people believe that CFS and fibromyalgia are two separate conditions, while others believe that the two conditions are the same – but symptoms can vary. Because there is no evidence of inflammation in the brain or spinal cord that is implied by the term encephalomyelitis, doctors tend to use the term CFS as the main symptom is generally fatigue and the condition is chronic (persistent).

While people with the condition tend to prefer the term ME as they may have other symptoms as well, they also feel the word fatigue does not reflect the severity of the fatigue that they have.

What Causes CFS?

The cause of CFS is unknown. Like fibromyalgia, there are several theories, including that it is triggered by:

1. A viral infection, such as glandular fever.
2. A hormone imbalance.
3. Emotional trauma, mental exhaustion, depression and stress.
4. Problems with the individual's immune system.
5. Genetic predisposition.
6. Traumatic events.

As with fibromyalgia, there is no cure for chronic fatigue syndrome (CFS) and treatments available focus on managing physical and emotional symptoms.

Common Symptoms of CFS

Some of the symptoms of CFS are the same as that of fibromyalgia. However, the primary symptom of CFS is extreme fatigue following physical or mental activity that does not go away with rest or sleep.

The flare-up of symptoms after exercise can be delayed for several hours or even until the next day. Generally, the ability to perform usual activities is affected. The feelings of fatigue are both physical and mental, and can be overwhelming. Sufferers report that the tiredness is different to anything they have previously experienced, and even after sleeping they do not feel refreshed. Other symptoms may include one or more of the following:

- severe headaches
- joint and muscular pain
- poor concentration and short-term memory/brain fog
- painful lymph nodes
- sensitivity to alcohol and certain foods
- problems similar to irritable bowel syndrome
- insomnia and lack of quality sleep
- sore throat
- sensitivity or intolerance to loud noise or light
- balance problems
- dizziness
- difficulty controlling body temperature
- irritability
- panic attacks
- depression.

CFS Diagnosis

CFS can take a long time to diagnose as there is no specific test available and other conditions that have similar symptoms must be ruled out first. NICE – The National Institute for Health and Clinical Excellence – state that doctors should consider a diagnosis of CFS if the patient is suffering from fatigue and all of the following apply:

- it is persistent and/or recurrent
- it is new or had a clear starting point (it has not been a lifelong problem)

- it is unexplained by other conditions
- it substantially reduces the amount of activity you can do
- it feels worse after physical activity.

The patient should also have one or more of these symptoms:

- insomnia or difficulty sleeping
- muscle or joint pain without inflammation (swelling)
- headaches
- painful lymph nodes that are not enlarged
- sore throat
- poor mental function, such as difficulty thinking
- symptoms worsening after physical or mental exertion
- feeling unwell or having flu-like symptoms
- nausea
- dizziness
- heart palpitations (without heart disease).

A clinician should confirm this diagnosis after other conditions have been ruled out, where the above symptoms have persisted for four months in an adult and three months in a child or young person.

Summary

As I am sure you have noticed, the similarities between fibromyalgia and CFS are easy to spot. Some doctors treat fibromyalgia (FMS) and chronic fatigue syndrome (CFS) separately, while others believe they are variations of the same condition. I was diagnosed with both conditions. This guide does not recommend the use of additional medication or invasive treatments; instead, it provides self-help treatments.

Part of my recovery was to stop describing myself as suffering from fibromyalgia/CFS. In the past I found myself telling people I met that I had fibromyalgia as a way of explaining my limping or tiredness.

Once I commenced my recovery programme, I deliberately gave no explanation. I recognised that fibromyalgia and CFS are just words. This label was not me and my condition did not define me. I chose to think of myself as someone whose body, mind and soul needed to be nurtured and allowed to relax in order to re-energise and renew.

PLEASE NOTE:

You should always seek medical advice and obtain a diagnosis from your medical practitioner to rule out any other conditions exhibiting similar symptoms. The information contained within this guide is for general purposes only.

Chapter Two – My Fibromyalgia/CFS Journey

Out of something bad comes something good.

Proverb.

Introduction

This story has a happy outcome. It is not about my life in general, but I think it may help you to know a bit about my personal story and what I did to recover.

> ☺ I am naturally a very private person, so it has been hard for me to share the details, but I feel it is important for you to understand my journey. If I can help just one person to achieve something good or beneficial from fibromyalgia/CFS, it will be worth it.

I am a really happy, positive person by nature, but there have been some very low points on my journey and many sufferers have found that they can identify with similarities in their own life. If at any stage of reading my story you become distressed about events in your life – please stop reading this chapter and go to the next one. That is where I start to share my methods for living in a very different way so that you can learn how to control and overcome fibromyalgia and/or CFS.

Rebecca's Story

My childhood was both difficult and traumatic, suffering poverty and abuse, and a whole heap of stress, throughout my twenties and thirties. With good reason I was often scared and worried, but I was raised to get on with things and not to feel sorry for myself – no matter how bad things got. I learnt to cope with whatever life brought my way, kept quiet about it and considered myself lucky! I distinctly remember that whenever I got overtired or distressed, my legs would ache and at the time I was told it was growing pains. I cannot be sure that it was connected to my fibromyalgia (FMS), but research suggests that this type of childhood pain could be the early onset of the condition.

From the day I left school at sixteen I was determined to escape from poverty and create a better life for myself. I worked very long hours and attended college in the evenings. It was not uncommon for me to work over seventy hours per week.

I passed all my professional exams and embarked on my career. Although work was enjoyable and financially rewarding, it came with heaps of stress and anxiety, on top of all my childhood issues that were still locked away in the cupboard of my mind.

Much of my life was an intense medley of work, tension and trauma. I would wake up every day feeling happy for the first few seconds and then worry would overwhelm me as I recalled the reality of my life. I would feel physically sick and whilst it was a situation of my own making, as is often the case with people who have problems, I felt completely trapped. I pressed on, dealing with things and getting on with my life, without seeking professional help and feeling completely isolated. Rarely did I relax. I was constantly so stressed out that I had pains in my chest – but still I kept on going.

Most days I was so tired I would go to bed at 9.00 p.m. so I could cope with the demands of the next day. During this time I suffered from occasional bouts of pain in my arms and legs, but guess what? – I ignored them.

Throughout this period of my life I had incredibly low self-esteem and I disliked myself intensely. No matter how much success I achieved, it did nothing to increase my feelings of self-worth.

I got married at twenty, but it soon became apparent that we were not right for each other, both being completely unable to meet the other's needs. Then in 1992, my daughter was born. So now there was another person to worry about – but what a person! What wouldn't I do for my adorable daughter? To touch her tiny hand, to look into her rich brown eyes, to hear her gurgle and then the clincher: her tiny laugh that made my life complete.

When I was with her things were great and I wanted to be with her every moment of every day. But like most people I couldn't, because it was my career that provided the essentials in life. Very soon I resented my job, because it stopped me from being with my daughter. But at the same time I knew it was a necessary evil if I was to avoid putting her through the poverty I had experienced in my own childhood. I felt I was letting her down. She was so innocent and made me so happy and yet I wasn't there for her. How do you explain to a child that mummy loves her but that she cannot be with her today?

The final blow was when I realised my marriage was over. So now it was just my baby and me ... only by this stage I had a complete lack of energy and experienced frequent fibromyalgia/CFS attacks. Now, I had different stresses to contend with as a single mum working full-time. Thankfully, I earned good money; although it was still a challenge holding everything together and I was exhausted. In many ways I had a lot to be thankful for; indeed, more than most. But there was only one thing I really wanted: to be a full-time mum and to make sure that my daughter had a better childhood than I did.

Her childminder was amazing (one of my wonderful sisters) and whilst I knew that she was getting all the love and attention she needed, I still had this strong urge inside me to be with her – she was the only important thing in my life. Every day it hurt knowing I couldn't be with her as much as I wanted and the pain in my limbs increasingly debilitated me.

Somehow, I managed to get through the days and even advance my career. I would relish precious moments with my daughter before going to work and again in the evening. She would be bathed and in bed, having been read a story, by 7.00 p.m. each night. When she was asleep I was left alone to brood over the pains and stresses in my life and I would be in bed early most nights. I was so stressed out that even though I was exhausted, sleep eluded me. I would lie there praying for help to be a good mum, agonising over what I could do to resolve my issues. Hours later I would slip into a fitful sleep, waking feeling like I had not been to sleep at all.

In 1998, I finally got my life on track when I married my second husband. Life was definitely better and I felt happier and more secure than ever. There was still plenty of stress in my hectic and rapidly progressing career, which meant living life at a fast pace. Coping with a career and being a wife, mum and stepmum while my husband worked away during the week was not easy. I also had the added stress of helping my husband deal with the aftermath of his divorce – and with it a lack of money and other external factors that threatened our happiness. Fortunately, we were both totally focused on loving each other and protecting our children. No matter what was thrown at us, no matter how much pain it caused us, we always put the needs of our children first, even if it meant more pain or difficulties for us.

> ☺ For the first time in my life I felt loved. I realised that I was a worthwhile person and that there was no reason to hate myself.

With a large family of two adults and five children, including my stepchildren, it was a struggle to maintain a work–life balance. Whilst my husband worked hard to provide for us all we still needed two incomes, as is the case with most families these days.

Despite focusing all my attention on my daughter when I was home, I still felt guilty that I could not be there for her all of the time. And despite working when she was in bed to keep on top of my workload, I then felt guilty that I was not giving enough attention to my job. I didn't seem to be able to do either justice.

My conditions finally became overwhelming and incapacitating in 1999. I had been diagnosed with osteoarthritis in my hands, which was extremely painful and becoming increasingly so. Apparently, I was about ten years too young to have developed it. Then I went through a period of approximately four months when I kept thinking I had the flu, although without all of the symptoms. I was constantly exhausted and I ached all over. Then it would go away for a few weeks, only to return worse than ever.

Strangely, whenever I did relax properly, for example at weekends or at Christmas, I felt really unwell. I would come in from work and practically collapse. I was desperate to spend time with my daughter and new husband, but often this would mean lying on the couch together watching a Disney movie while I struggled to stay awake.

> ☺ I came up with what I thought was a great idea to help me relax: I took sugarcraft classes once a week with my sister. We did have a good laugh but guess what – it ended up being stressful because we took professional exams and I would be up at 5.00 a.m. icing cakes before my daughter got up. Are you beginning to get the impression I was not great at relaxing?!

My symptoms became progressively worse. The attacks lasted longer, they were increasingly severe and they became more and more frequent. I have always been very fit – I joined my first gym at sixteen, so exercise has always been an important part of my life – but by this stage things had got so bad that I could barely move. I was a member of a fitness club at the time and my daughter went come with me.

The changing rooms were on the ground floor but the gym was on the first floor and eventually I could not even get up the stairs, never mind exercise. By this time the pain was incessant and I had all of the symptoms at least five days of every week. I had a company car yet I did not feel safe enough to drive to work, so I arranged for someone to collect me.

Looking back, I must have been constantly running on adrenaline, because as soon as I relaxed I felt like I had been hit by a truck. At the time I still worked in a very stressful environment and would arrive at work feeling like I was about to collapse, but within an hour the adrenaline would kick in and I could just about manage to cope until the end of the working day. I realised this was no way to live, but at the time I couldn't see a way out – I was allowing myself to feel trapped.

☺ The pain never totally disappeared and I would limp around a bit like the hero in an action movie, but at least I would make it through the day.

By now not only was I physically impaired, but I was also becoming increasingly worried about memory and my ability to think clearly. I actually felt embarrassed about this because I didn't know what was wrong with me and I felt inadequate because it was so unlike me. I struggled even with basic things and as I was a senior manager, leading a large team, I was worried about people finding out. I had always been able to take in large amounts of information very quickly and clarify difficult topics with ease, but these skills were rapidly disappearing. I knew I needed to give up work and yet we had a mortgage and bills to pay, and a family to support.

It was shortly after this that I saw a consultant, who diagnosed me with fibromyalgia/CFS and explained how stress aggravates the condition. He told me that if I didn't change my lifestyle, I would end up in a wheelchair …

☺ This was a turning point in my life. I was so scared that I knew I had to take positive action.

I resigned from my highly paid job the very next day and took a position working for twenty-one hours a week for a less dynamic organisation. Fortunately, they were very understanding about the fact that I needed less stress. I changed my personal life also and made things easier at home by employing a lovely lady for eighteen hours a week to help around the house. She did everything apart from the cooking. I felt bad that I had to rely on someone thirty years older than me to keep the house going, but she was happy to have the work and I really thought I had solved the problem.

I was far less stressed and actually went through a period of semi-remission for a few months. I was by no means symptom-free, but the attacks were certainly less frequent, maybe once or twice a week, as I was getting lots of rest. Then the company underwent a management reshuffle. The leadership team changed and with it my stress levels and workload began to creep up again, as did the symptoms. They were actually worse than ever before.

My Symptoms

1. Exhaustion

I was completely exhausted physically almost all of the time and I literally dreaded receiving an invitation to family or social events, being unable to stay up after 9.00 p.m. Before I was diagnosed I found this really embarrassing and I was convinced everyone would think I was a complete misery; at least afterwards I had a label I could use to explain my condition. However, the problem with labels is that it can become your identity and you gradually become more of what you understand the label means.

My exhaustion made me irritable and difficult to live with. I often remember wanting to shout at my husband if he delayed me from sitting down because he wanted a hug. I knew he was just being his usual loving self, but in my head I would be screaming: Are you stupid? Don't you know how bad I feel? I don't need a hug – I need to lie down.

☺ I don't think I ever actually said it out loud (well maybe once or twice), but that didn't make me feel any less guilty.

2. Sleep problems

I struggled to get to sleep because of the pain and would wake up frequently. I had to change position throughout the night in an effort to make my neck comfortable. But with the other tender points to contend with there was really no comfortable position to sleep in, because wherever these points made contact with the mattress it was extremely painful. I would also know about it if my husband moved while we were in bed and accidentally touched my elbow, for example.

In the morning I would wake up feeling like I had been trampled by elephants. I couldn't face having to get up and function as a normal human being, which meant that I couldn't live a normal life as such. I remember thinking some mornings that I should be in hospital and that no one this unwell should be left to suffer in silence. My exhaustion meant that I used to feel nauseous, but I knew that if I slept it would ease off; it was a vicious circle.

3. Pain

Both my muscles and limbs ached and burned, but it was unlike any pain I had ever experienced from exercise – it was far more intense, as though my nerve endings were on fire. Painkillers had no effect, which in itself was really frustrating.

4. Tender points

I had seventeen of the eighteen known tender points recognised as the criteria used for classification (of a minimum of eleven), which meant that basic things people take for granted such as sitting or lying down were really uncomfortable. Yet, it was these things that I really needed to do, owing to the complete and utter exhaustion, and the discomfort I felt.

☺ Actually, I had all eighteen, but one was not as tender as the rest – note: this is me focusing on the positives.

5. Muscle spasms/twitches

My muscles often went into spasm and twitched beyond my control. These sensations were extremely strange, annoying and unpleasant and whilst they only lasted a few seconds, I often found myself crying out in pain.

6. Sore skin

I could not bear for anyone, including my daughter or husband, to touch me. The sensation was a bit like having sunburn and someone hugging you. I felt so guilty about wanting to push them away whenever they put their arms around me to give me a cuddle. I needed my husband to hold me and make me feel safe, but at the same time I couldn't let him because of how it made me feel. Forced to reject affection because I was so sore, love really did hurt.

7. Neck pain

My neck hurt like crazy and the pain was incessant. I used to roll up a towel and position it under my neck before going to sleep to try to alleviate the discomfort. Looking back, I realise now that I should have tried sleeping in a soft collar. But at the time the thought was too depressing and they are hardly attractive nightwear for a married woman!

I was unable to carry everyday things like bags without triggering pain in my neck that would be unbearable and continuous for days. Driving for more than fifteen minutes at a time was also impossible, because the pain would become so bad that it would reduce my concentration. I was also unable to support things for sustained periods for the same reason.

I would frequently wake up with excruciating neck pain, so much so that I literally could not move my head without being in agony. It was like an incessant burning sensation or ache rather than a throbbing. However, it was nonetheless incredibly intense and if I moved I would experience acute shooting pains. I knew that the only way to ease it was to move my head, so I would stand in the shower sobbing whilst trying to move my head through the pain until it eased off slightly.

My husband was incredibly supportive during this time and he would help me out of bed in the morning and run the shower for me. Because I woke frequently at night he would check if I was OK. He was always very patient, even though he had to get up at 6.00 a.m., and I felt guilty about it.

8. Lack of concentration/brain (fibro) fog

I have always had a great memory and was fortunate enough to be able to both absorb information very quickly and retain it. So to get to the stage where I struggled to remember even basic things was incredibly demoralising. I thought I was losing my mind and constantly forgot what I was supposed to be doing. If I was reading I would forget what I had read and I used to forget the way to places – even places I had been to often. It never lasted long, in that my mind would just go blank for a few seconds, but it was frightening and frustrating nonetheless – sometimes dangerous.

9. Intense menstrual period pain

My body was so sensitive to pain that every month I dreaded my menstrual cycle because I knew I was going to be in agony. No amount of drugs or painkillers made any impact and neither did TENS machines or hot-water bottles. I became irritable and the fatigue was disabling.

10. Poor circulation

With the burning or tingling sensation, and the swelling in my hands and feet, my rings constantly got stuck and felt like they were cutting into my fingers, so most days I would not even be able to wear my wedding ring.

11. Feeling an urgent need to urinate

This was an incredibly distressing problem. I was back and forth from the toilet all the time because of the overstimulated nerve endings in the bladder, sometimes within minutes of sitting down. And if I didn't go, then because of my increased sensitivity to pain, it became excruciating. The only way I could cope with long journeys or meetings where I would not be able to get up or leave to go to the toilet was to avoid drinking and pray.

With each month the attacks got worse and lasted longer and longer, until it seemed the symptoms were permanent. I tried all sorts of remedies including acupuncture, prescribed medication and supplements. The acupuncture brought some relief to the pain in my knees, but nothing made any real difference. I took two months off work, but there was no improvement.

☺ Thankfully, my husband took charge – not that I was in a position to argue, as I was exhausted and just wanted to be looked after. We ate meals that were easy to prepare or he cooked. Despite our worries over money, he made me resign from my part-time job and we moved away from the city to a small village in the countryside. He let me think it over for all of thirty seconds, provided I agreed!

I was optimistic in nature and believed wholeheartedly that this would be the cure, the answer to all of our problems. I would relax for a year, giving my body the opportunity to recover, and then get back to normal. However, this gave me plenty of time on my hands and the symptoms remained as long as I continued to analyse them.

For four years I lived a restricted life, resting for most of the day while my husband was working long hours and my daughter was at school. I did everything I could to avoid stressful situations and to allow my body to recover, but nothing seemed to make much difference.

Through sheer determination, I reached a point where I could walk my daughter to school – provided I rested afterwards. On good days I was able to drive short distances. I learnt to push myself through the pain in order to do things that I wanted achieve, but I would suffer the consequences for days afterwards.

I am sure you have heard the expression 'be careful what you wish for'. I had spent years longing to be a stay-at-home mum because I thought it would make me a better mum. Now, I had been granted my wish. Yet, despite the fact that I was at home all the time, my condition meant it was a constant struggle for me to be the kind of mum I wanted to be.

During this time I learnt to paint in watercolours, but on bad days I could not even hold the paintbrush because both my arms and neck ached. Neither could I read most days because I found holding a book for any length of time too tiring and painful, never mind turning the pages.

I felt completely isolated and extremely low. No matter how much people tried and how nice they were, I knew that they did not understand. To them, I looked completely healthy on the outside and so they were unable to appreciate the feelings of isolation, frustration, loneliness and guilt that go with this condition, unless they had suffered from it themselves.

My symptoms got increasingly worse and I became more and more withdrawn, until one day a very dear friend described me as having retired from life!

> ☺ Writing these paragraphs reminds me of how bad it was, but it is important that you know the details and take faith in the fact that you, too, can recover from this debilitating illness or at least cope and learn to manage this condition. The agonies of these moments became the driving force behind the positive changes I created in order to escape from the endless agony and lack of energy. I will share my methods in later chapters to help you regain your life and have a great future.

After three years of resting I managed to feel less stressed and because I was desperate to be so-called normal, I would push myself to do normal things with my family and friends. Afterwards, I would know about it and I would be forced to spend days lying on the couch in agony.

Then at a routine check-up my doctor told me about a special pain clinic for fibromyalgia (FMS) and ME/CFS and asked if I wanted to attend a course of treatment there. It was half an hour's drive away, so my husband and I agreed that he would take me if I was ever too tired to drive; we could not miss out on this opportunity and I had to do something if I was to recover.

> ☺ He actually ended up driving me to all of the sessions and never once made me feel guilty that he would have to catch up on work or was giving up his holidays – honestly, the man is a saint!

The clinic was run by a clinical psychologist who explained how the way we think affects our condition and the way we feel physically. It was there that I began my journey into the power of the mind, overcoming my exhaustion and pain, and regaining my health.

At the clinic we were asked to go into a very detailed analysis of how much energy we used on daily activities. It even included low-energy activities such as having a conversation. For weeks we monitored the effects our activities had on our symptoms. I found this period of my life very depressing, because it made me focus on how pathetic my life was and how little I could actually do. But at the same time I could see the sense in what he was saying.

> ☺ I am eternally grateful to the team at the clinic as they explained how the way we think and our mood affect the way we feel. I will never forget sitting in that group. There were about fourteen of us and I remember listening to other people insisting they had no control over their body or their symptoms.
>
> This is where our differences lay, for inside I was jumping for joy. It became apparent that I was the only one who felt this way. But part of me was determined to be different and believe it was possible to get better. Yes, I thought, maybe I could finally find a way to control this terrible illness.

It was at this point that I began to learn more about the power of the unconscious mind. I read lots of books and focused on putting the methods into practise. Initially it was very difficult for me to read, because by the time I got to the bottom of the page I had forgotten what I had just read. To overcome this I gave myself lots of breaks to rest my mind, arms and neck. Wherever possible I got audio books, but eventually it got easier and my fibro (brain) fog began to clear as I became more and more engrossed in studying the power of the mind and the mind–body connection.

Gradually I started to feel better, which spurred me on even more. I studied several courses and trained in various therapies, gaining qualifications in Time Line Therapy™, hypnosis, coaching and NLP (Neuro Linguistic Programming). Everything I learnt, I adapted to my illness and I worked on myself constantly. I was beginning to feel great and my flare-ups became milder and less frequent, until one day they disappeared altogether! In the following chapters I will be sharing all of these techniques with you so that you might begin to work on your own self and change your own life or view, too.

At the same time, whilst I put my all into it and for the first time in years felt I was beginning to recover, I was sensible and made sure I did not overdo things. I told myself I needed six months before I could be completely reassured that it was gone.

It is my belief that stress greatly contributed to all of my symptoms, including the amount of pain I felt. In the back of my mind, I was concerned about what would happen if I encountered a stressful situation. I knew I was now equipped to control my condition, pain, wellness, anxieties and stress, but inside I still had a niggling doubt. Was I in control or could the stress overwhelm me again? Then my first big challenge came.

We had moved into another house to help one of our children get on the property ladder and were in the middle of a massive renovation project, whilst still living in the property. The whole project was meant to take six months, but after this period we were less than a third of the way through the work. Our builder seemed unable to finish the job for whatever reason; we had no heating, kitchen or proper bathroom and his only other worker had been assigned another job. Only half the property had a roof, the back half of the house had no walls and most rooms had water leaking in. We were unable to cook proper meals and our clothes and furniture were mouldy because of the damp. Actually, it was even worse than I have described, but I am sure you will have got the general idea. Costs were escalating and we stood to lose tens of thousands of pounds – it was a very difficult time.

It was now late 2006 and I had begun focusing on total healing. We had been in our new 'house' for twelve months when I asked my unconscious mind, God and the universe what I needed to know in order to live a healthy life until the age of 97.

I had the symptoms of a bladder infection two weeks later after setting my goal of reaching the age of 97, but the urine test proved negative. About a month later it came back, but again the test was negative. So my GP sent me for an ultrasound scan, 'just to see if my tubes were twisted'. My tubes were fine, but the ultrasound showed a growth in my left kidney. They believed it to be an angiomyolipoma (a rare, well-known soft tissue tumour which is usually benign), but they booked me in for an MRI scan to make sure.

It was a few days after this that part of the roof fell in; the actual roof on the house, that is, not my world – I told you we had a poor builder. The universe then delivered a lovely man called Ernie, who took charge of the building project. He brought in a team of skilled workmen and craftsmen, who worked long hours to put our home back together.

The initial diagnosis proved correct and the growth in my kidney was, indeed, benign, but it would not have been responsible for causing the bladder infections. However, the MRI scan revealed an unidentified growth in my pancreas.

Statistics on the Internet revealed that only 3 per cent of people who have pancreatic cancer live for more than five years. I don't mind admitting I was terrified. Not because I was afraid of death but because I could not bear the thought of leaving my daughter and husband behind. I knew they would take care of each other, but I also knew how much they both needed me and the feeling was reciprocated.

I spent twenty-four hours lying in my husband's arms, planning what I would do if the news spelt the worst. Then my thoughts turned to the fact that I had asked my mind and my body to help me live a healthy life until the age of 97 and I put this process into overdrive; though I knew that this was just a small part of the procedure. My husband and I immediately organised an endoscopic scan to see what was going on inside, so that I could find out exactly what I had and to enable me to start to fight it.

We went to London three days before Christmas, where I had the scan, but they still could not ascertain what the tumour was. It was particularly emotional as we stood in front of the huge Christmas tree in Trafalgar Square, listening to the carols, yet the whole time my mind was focused on my healing techniques.

On Christmas Eve, the walls having been plastered just hours beforehand and the kitchen still only half finished, we put our tree up. By this time about half the house was just about habitable. I stood in front of our own tree and thought: no way is this going to be my last Christmas.

I had more than half my pancreas removed in February 2007, the day after my daughter's thirteenth birthday. Thankfully, I was calm and confident about the outcome and I spent the time in hospital whilst waiting for my operation and various tests to be completed painting watercolour postcards.

My husband and I had decided before the operation that since it was such a dangerous operation and because of what I had been told to expect afterwards, it wasn't something we wanted our daughter to see and I so I knew it would be at least a week before I was in any condition to see her. We sat on my hospital bed while she opened her presents and I hugged her and said, 'I'll see you in a week, princess. I promise you I'll be fine.' I meant every word.

> ☺ My surgeon told me that no previous pain – even that of fibromyalgia/CFS – could prepare me for the excruciating pain I would be in ... great!

I was booked in for a fifteen-hour Whipple operation. If you are not too squeamish – Google it! Thankfully, they did not need to remove my entire pancreas.

My surgeon was really not exaggerating about the pain. Despite the doctors providing me with extremely strong pain relief, there were two occasions in particular when the pain was unbearable. One was a couple of days after my operation, when the epidural I had been given to administer pain relief became disconnected. At the time I was advised that they could not increase the dosage, but of course what they and I did not realise was that none was getting through. The second time was the night before it was discovered I had contracted MRSA, when I was in excruciating pain from the nerve endings around my 25-centimetre scar, which was infected. On both occasions the doctors acted to administer pain relief as quickly as they could, but I was very grateful for the techniques in this book while waiting for them to take effect.

Despite contracting a life-threatening MRSA infection whilst I was in hospital, I made a quick recovery. I had made myself hypnosis CDs beforehand and worked through lots of healing processes. It was while I was still recovering from MRSA that I looked at a small pink freckle that I'd had on my arm for years and thought: I won't feel safe until that's gone. It was a strange thought to have, having not yet received the results of the biopsy on my tumour. As it turned out, the tumour was apparently very rare and the surgeon told me I had been incredibly lucky, as it was still benign but was of a type that usually turned malignant.

A month after I came out of hospital I saw my GP about the freckle and was assured it was nothing. I knew from research I had done that it did not look like a malignant melanoma and it had not changed in appearance, but my mind kept telling me I had to get it checked out by a specialist.

I was back at the doctors a month later, only this time I was sent to the hospital – more to put my mind at rest rather than because something was actually wrong. The surgeon assured me it was nothing and that it had none of the usual characteristics of a malignant melanoma, but she agreed to remove it nonetheless to stop me from worrying. Once the biopsy was done I was told would receive a letter in two weeks to confirm all was well.

About ten days later a call came asking me to attend the hospital that same day. I remember the surgeon saying to me, 'Thank God you know your own body.' It was a malignant melanoma, caught in the very early stages but only weeks away from being stage II skin cancer.

Thankfully, I have made a full recovery from both conditions. I do not have any ongoing treatments and despite having less than half my pancreas, I am not diabetic. Although I will be monitored for the rest of my life, I am confident I will reach a ripe old age.

☺ Throughout this time my fibromyalgia/CFS did not flare up. Today, I remain in control of it – it no longer controls me. In fact, I am fitter now than ever and I lead a fantastic life.

When I was discharged from hospital I was supplied with masses of extremely strong painkillers, but I did not use any and later took them back to my local chemist to be disposed of – I had my own methods of dealing with the pain.

Of course I do experience pain, like everyone else. In fact, it would be highly dangerous not to feel pain – how else would I know if I were touching something too hot, grasping a sharp blade too tightly, or that I had an illness or injury of some sort?

Summary

I am now able to live a normal life and I am truly happy. My positivity is infectious and people describe me as having an energy that makes them feel positive and safe. These days I am able to work again as an author, publisher and book writing coach. I am very fit once more and I am able to exercise five or six times a week.

My life so far has certainly been eventful and challenging, but I feel very fortunate because my journey has brought me to a great place and equipped me with skills that will enable me to flourish. Not only am I symptom-free, but I also have what I call 'emotional balance'. I love my work – writing and coaching others is very satisfying. My personal life is fantastic and I am really happy with who I am. I feel complete and worthy of the wonderful life I am privileged to lead.

It is my great pleasure to share my techniques with you and give you the opportunity to regain control of your life. Let's now begin your journey ... and if you choose to adopt my approach, I sincerely hope that it will work for you as well as it does for me.

Chapter Three – The Awesome Power of the Mind

It is better to light one small candle than curse the darkness.

Chinese Proverb

Introduction

Your mind is the most powerful computer on the planet and your software is what controls your behaviour and thinking. Even though your brain is efficient and complex, it is actually relatively simple to understand, because there are only two ways you make sense of your world: consciously and unconsciously.

Understanding how your mind works is the first step to unlocking its potential. Don't panic – I am not going to ask you to become a professor of neurology. I am simply suggesting that you increase your understanding of how you make sense of your world, both consciously and unconsciously.

When I first learnt the information I am about to share with you, it was a revelation. Suddenly, so many things from my past that I had long tried and failed to make sense of became easier to understand.

In turn, my present experiences became more enjoyable, productive and rewarding.

Your Conscious Mind

This is the section of your mind with which you think deliberately – it is where decision-making takes place. While this is the part of your thinking you are consciously aware of, research shows that it can only retain a handful of ideas at any one time.

> ☺ Yes, I know some of you, like me, will be great at multitasking – I even used to study whilst watching television and still pass my exams – but as you will discover later, it is not a great idea.

No matter how hard you try, you cannot think about several things at the same time. But you might be able to engage in one activity that you no longer have to focus on consciously – like washing the dishes – whilst thinking about another thing, such as how you are going to pay the mortgage this month. This is because the unconscious part of the mind has taken over one of the tasks, leaving you free to think about or worry about something else.

Your Unconscious Mind

Your unconscious mind is the largest section of your mind and it receives and processes millions of bits of information every second via your senses:

- visual – sight
- auditory – hearing
- kinaesthetic – touch and movement
- gustatory – taste
- olfactory – smell

If it processed all of this information so that you were aware of it consciously, it would be too much for you to cope with, so it filters the information down to about 140 pieces. This means that your brain could focus on your symptoms and delete other information.

For instance, until you read this you were probably not aware of the feeling of your shoe on your left foot or which parts of your body were not hurting.

Your unconscious mind contains all of your memories and may even repress some painful ones. When you are asleep your conscious mind is resting, but your unconscious mind continues to carry out many functions, including dreaming, as it helps you process what has happened during the day.

I often hear people say they had a really weird dream last night and don't know why. But I think it is relatively simple to trace the origin of most of my dreams. If I have had a dream, I break down all of the elements and on almost all occasions, I am able to match these to fleeting thoughts I have had during the day. For example, I recently had a dream where I was running through a river of ice cream and then suddenly I was trying on a furry black-and-white dress (not my usual style☺), while trying to push the buttons on a machine to save the world.

Crazy, perhaps – but more likely it was because during the day, while dashing through a local shopping centre, I had glanced over at an ice-cream shop that sold twenty flavours and fleetingly thought how lovely they looked. I would also have given passing thoughts to some of the clothes I had seen. Then later in the day my husband, knowing my love of animals, mentioned that they were planning to get a pair of pandas at Edinburgh Zoo. That evening, I watched an episode of *Lost* – and if you have ever seen it, you will understand where the last aspect of the dream came from. In my opinion dreams are the unconscious mind's way of dealing with thoughts and events of the day and in effect filing them – an essential part of the sleep process.

> A good laugh and a long sleep are the best cures in the doctor's book.
>
> Irish Proverb

I often forget about a dilemma, confident that within an hour or so of waking up I will have a solution. That is because the unconscious mind has the ability to help you process solutions while you sleep. One very important task of the unconscious mind is that it holds the blueprint for perfect health. If you are having trouble accepting this, ask yourself which part of your mind keeps you alive whilst you are asleep.

Most of our habits function in the unconscious mind. Whenever we learn to do something, it becomes automated over time and so we become unconsciously skilled at it. As well as useful skills like tying shoelaces, driving a car and washing our hair, we can also become unconsciously skilled at thought processes – including making ourselves feel happy, depressed or anxious. Even focusing on pain can become an unconscious habit.

Understanding that your thoughts are not facts and that you can retrain your brain to change the way you experience illness can be a difficult concept to grasp. However, once you understand how your brain is interpreting the information it receives via your five senses and incorporate this knowledge using my techniques, you can begin to manage your fibromyalgia/CFS.

We live in a world where technology is advancing so quickly many of us struggle to keep up. Frequently, new gadgets come with an enormous range of features and often they only include a very basic user guide. We are then expected to go online to get full details of how to get the most out of the product's features. Some people don't bother doing this and try guessing how to use the various functions, perhaps asking someone they know who has a similar piece of equipment.

The brain is far more complex than even the most advanced gadgets available and we are all born without an instruction manual. The only instructions we receive during our lifetime are from our parents, teachers, siblings and peers. So we don't actually have any instructions, really, and certainly not a comprehensive list. We only know what other people pass on to us and if they are doing something the hard way, then that is the way they show us how to do it, too. But we are only human and we make mistakes – and hopefully learn from them.

Many people go through their entire life feeling like they have no control over their thinking or behaviour. My new clients frequently make statements like: 'It's just the way I am' or 'I'm the kind of person who will always ...' But the fact is we are not our behaviours or the way we think. We can learn to change both the way we think and the way we behave in any way we wish.

If you are positive about your ability to overcome your illness, the quicker and more effective your results will be. As the American industrialist Henry Ford famously said: 'Whether you think you can, or think you can't, you're probably right.'

That said, if you are not convinced – don't give up. Putting this book on a shelf (shelf therapy) and not even finishing it will certainly not help you. There are processes in this guide that will start to take effect within a few days and once you begin to make progress, it will spur you on to use the other techniques. The key is to practise, practise, practise.

Fibromyalgia and CFS are not illnesses of the mind but, as with many other illnesses, how you think and feel has a direct impact on your condition. Recently, someone told me that it made her feel weak-minded that she had not been able to think herself out of her symptoms. This is not the case at all. You cannot just think your symptoms away. But I do believe that, like me, once you understand the techniques available, you can use them to gain freedom from your symptoms forever.

Many fibromyalgia/CFS sufferers do not like to accept that their feelings have any bearing on their illness, but I firmly believe the brain is key to managing symptoms. Fibromyalgia and CFS are no different to any other illnesses in that recovery is quicker in patients with a positive mental attitude.

When I was recovering from my pancreatectomy I had a very positive mindset and used various hypnosis sessions I had recorded to aid my healing. I was actually told by my specialist Macmillan nurse that I was making the fastest recovery in history. So in my opinion, using the mind to help me recover from fibromyalgia/CFS was no exception.

The Power of Hypnosis and Deep Relaxation

Hypnosis is a recognised technique frequently used to help people make changes in their behaviour and thinking. It is also used to overcome illness, particularly when related to the nervous system. This is why I believe it is so effective for fibromyalgia/CFS sufferers, as it enables the unconscious mind to desensitise the ability to feel pain. Hypnosis is a therapeutic practice that is designed to create an altered state of consciousness in order to stimulate the body and mind to relax deeply, thereby enabling the unconscious mind to become more suggestible.

It is generally accepted that all hypnosis is ultimately self-hypnosis. A hypnotist merely helps to facilitate your experience – it is about empowerment. During a hypnotherapy session you do not lose control. You are not unconscious, you cannot 'get stuck' in hypnosis and you are not made to do anything you do not wish to do. So despite what you see to the contrary in movies or on television, it is not possible to make you do something under hypnosis that you would not otherwise want to do. In other words, no one can get you to rob a bank or anything like that.

Hypnosis is scientifically proven to be effective in creating change in certain repetitive behaviours, including quitting smoking as well as helping with weight loss, stress reduction, motivation and pain control. To discern hypnosis, it is first important to ascertain what it is not:

- sleeping
- unconsciousness in the sense of insensibility
- that you are gullible or easily deceived
- being weak-minded, impressionable or irresolute
- being controlled by someone else
- merely a gimmick for entertainment
- a loss of self-discipline or self-restraint.

As part of my journey into the power of the mind I studied to become a master practitioner of hypnosis. And within this guide I have shared techniques that will allow you to become more relaxed, change your thinking and behaviour, and in turn gain better sleep. To aid my recovery I knew I needed to relax deeply so that I could speak to my body and allow it to heal and recover.

To do this I recorded three wonderful hypnosis sessions that I could replay over and over to myself whenever needed:

- one was a wonderful energising start to each day in a positive light;
- the second was a powerful healing session;
- the third was a beautiful relaxation filled with gratitude, to allow me to end the day and fall asleep from a very good place.

If you decide to use the services of a hypnotherapist, conduct your research first. Make sure they are reputable, that they understand fibromyalgia/CFS and you are comfortable with them. Alternatively, there is a range of pre-recorded hypnosis and relaxation products available on the market that may prove to be more cost-effective and convenient.

Hypnosis that targets fibromyalgia/CFS specifically is the most effective, but a general deep-relaxation CD may be just as effective for some people. For details of my personal sessions, please visit: <www.forgetfibromyalgia.com>.

Perception

Our perception of everything we experience is based on our beliefs and values. The way in which we perceive something explains why two people can experience the same event, yet have a completely different view of it. For example, take two people who have very different beliefs and values about what a relaxing evening entails. For one person the ideal way to spend their time might be with a large group of friends on a night out on the town. Whereas the other might regard this as a nightmare, preferring to relax with a book in the company of a loved one. It is our beliefs, values and thoughts that create our emotions – not the external event. We all experience an external event, have thoughts based on our beliefs and values, then experience the emotion.

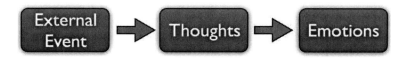

Perception is our personal opinion or viewpoint about any particular event. How we become aware of happiness, friendships, love, success, failure and in fact everything is just a perception. One day a client of mine spent the first ten minutes of her session telling me about something her father's new wife had done which she felt proved her stepmother hated her. When I explained that it was all about how she perceived the situation, she became angry, to the degree that she was close to tears and asked, 'So what you are saying is that it's my fault and I imagined it all.'

That was not what I was saying at all, but the fact remains that how we perceive things changes the event in our minds. Of course the event is fact, not imagination, but at the same time the reality is changed as it is filtered according to our beliefs and values. When I went on to give my client four different thoughts or intentions her stepmother could have had in relation to the same event, she was shocked, because she had never even considered that perhaps it had not been intended in the way she had interpreted the action. In fact, the following week she was able to report that one of my suggestions had been spot on!

During my corporate career I was made redundant twice – an event most people would find stressful. The first time happened at a particularly inconvenient time as we had just purchased our first home, when the company I worked for was sold and our entire division shut down. I was offered a role at the new head office, but that was 150 miles away from my new home. I was given three months' notice and saw it as a good opportunity. During that time I managed to secure three job offers and left with a good settlement, a big bonus and a new role in a new company, starting with immediate effect. So this experience for me was extremely positive.

Several years later during the restructure of another company I was working for at the time, everyone became very distressed at the prospect of redundancy. I, on the other hand, viewed the possibility as positive. So despite the offer of a new role I actually opted for redundancy, once again leaving with a settlement. Although I did not have a new job to go to at the time, I managed to secure a far more senior role in a larger company within two weeks. As this demonstrates, how we perceive any particular situation makes all the difference to how we react to it and therefore the subsequent events.

Because our perception is like wearing a pair of glasses to see things clearer, the glasses need to be of the correct prescription. At lunch recently with my three sisters we all tried on each other's reading glasses and as you might expect, found them completely unsuitable. Not surprisingly, as the youngest, I had the weakest prescription and they increased with the age of each sister.

> ☺ So next time you are reacting to something
> in a negative or unrealistic way, ask yourself if
> you are wearing the correct glasses.

There is no doubt that your current mood changes your perception, which some days makes you feel like everything is wrong or gives you that sense of 'impending-doom syndrome'. Your emotions – fear, anger, anxiety, happiness, joy and guilt – are a direct result of your internal processing that day, so it is no good blaming the weather, the event, the company, another person or even the government.

Your emotions follow your thoughts. You are the only person who is in charge of your feelings and emotions. Whenever you catch yourself starting to feel an inappropriate 'emotion', ask yourself: Does the way I am feeling really fit this situation? The more depressed or miserable you are feeling, the more negative you are going to feel about the events of that day.

Perceiving an event from another's viewpoint can be helpful. Ask yourself how a more positive you, or an optimistic friend, might react to the same event. If you are reacting badly to events, accept that it may just be because of the emotional state you are in that day and not necessarily that the event is so terrible.

We all experience life differently. By this I am not referring to the actual events that take place in our lives but how we interpret those events. In fact, we all live in our own unique world. As I explained earlier, our minds receive millions of bits of information every second. If we were aware of all the information we were receiving, our minds would be overloaded. So our unconscious mind does three things with the information it receives: deletes, distorts and generalises.

1. Deletion

Your mind deletes information it doesn't think is important at the time and brings to your attention things it thinks you do want to know. For instance, you were probably not conscious of the clothes on your body until you read this. Have you ever noticed that when you choose a new type of car you want that you see them everywhere? If you work for a company selling a particular sports brand, you will find that you constantly notice the type of trainers people are wearing.

> ☺ This is why children are able to completely delete all the toys, clothes, etc., scattered all over their bedrooms and be convinced they have tidied up!

2. Distortion

We all have our own unique model of the world. By this I mean that we all have beliefs and values that have been created over our lifetime – many of which stem from childhood – that affect our thinking and behaviour.

During childhood you were constantly learning and developing, so it makes perfect sense that your beliefs and values will have been developing, too. As they do so, they are greatly influenced by significant people in your life. If you think about your most important beliefs, it is generally possible to pinpoint which person you modelled or copied them from.

Our beliefs and values underpin everything we do. Some beliefs and values form through experience and again, it can be possible to identify events and experiences that led to a particular belief. When my clients have a belief that is adversely affecting their lives, they often find it easier to change that belief once they have identified the source.

Have you ever wondered why some people behave in a way that is totally unacceptable in your opinion, yet they think it is the correct way to behave? This is because they have very different beliefs and values to you, which as explained earlier means they perceive the event differently.

Your unconscious mind stores your beliefs and values and will actively seek out information that supports them. So if you are the type of person who believes that most people are bad and dishonest, or that everything goes wrong for you, you will tend to notice evidence that supports this.

☺ Or if, like me, you choose to believe that most people are kind, good and honest, you will find your world is filled with these people.

3. Generalisation

Your unconscious mind generalises information it receives, which is really useful because without this process, every time you came to a door you would have to work out how to open it. When it is less helpful is when you generalise events and categorise them as negative. For example, if you automatically assume that every time the phone rings it will be bad news or a problem, it will not be long before you dread the sound of the phone ringing.

For several years when my husband and I felt that our happiness and that of those we loved the most was under constant threat, I even dreaded the post arriving. Eventually, it invoked a physical reaction in that I felt ill and sick – not really a great way to start each day!

I noticed that gradually, over the years when I was suffering from fibromyalgia/CFS, I attributed more and more ailments to my condition and worried that it meant I was getting worse. It was an important part of my recovery process to acknowledge that healthy people get viruses and aches and pains as well, and that not everything I felt was related to fibromyalgia/CFS. Although I felt that my condition made everything feel worse, I realised that this was because I was so obsessed with checking my body for new symptoms and ailments that I was increasing the intensity of them.

Cause and Effect

Around 80 per cent of people live their lives near to or on the effect side of life. This means they feel that things happen to them and that they have no control over events. We all know people who feel like this and they are easy to spot by the things they say: I would be slim if it were not for my wife and the meals she cooks; I would have more money if it were not for the economy; my kids make me stressed. People who feel like this are not weak, but have given away their power, making them feel helpless. They have become victims of circumstances.

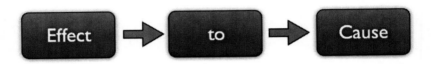

When people are at the cause side of life, they accept that most things in life have happened as a result of conscious or unconscious decisions they have made. Even when they genuinely feel that an event was outside their control, they recognise that while they may not always be able to control the events that come into their life, they *can* control how they react to them. They know that they are the pilot of their lives, that they are in charge of their brain and therefore the results they achieve.

Taking responsibility for your life is not about blaming yourself for mistakes or negative events, because this is also being a victim – a victim of yourself. So if you are the kind of person who thinks things like, I've messed up again, I'm such an idiot, then stop right now and accept that you were doing the best you could with the resources you had available at the time. A very good indicator of whether or not you are living close to the effect side of life is to ask yourself if you are feeling trapped.

People feel trapped when they cannot see a way out of a particular situation and when they believe they have no options. This way of thinking is guaranteed to make them feel helpless, frustrated or angry.

This is often the case with my clients and one lady in particular felt completely trapped in her marriage. She was desperately unhappy and resented everything her husband did, feeling as though he was her jailer. After a few sessions she realised that she was not actually trapped at all. Ending her marriage would have an effect on her life in that she would have had to live in a smaller house and manage her career whilst being a single parent, but it was feasible. When she acknowledged that her children did not have to suffer a traumatic divorce if both parents worked together for their long-term happiness, she no longer felt trapped. Once she realised she was not trapped, her feelings for her husband began to change, their relationship improved greatly and she no longer wanted to end their marriage.

Never Give Up

One of the biggest examples of something physical that people have to get through is recovering from an operation. It is difficult because after they have got through whatever medical procedure it was, they then have to go through the rehabilitation process of recovering from the procedure and the medical condition it was treating.

After my pancreatectomy I had an incredibly large wound called a rooftop, which meant that my mobility was impaired. The nurses were wonderful and they encouraged me to get up within a couple of days. I did really well, listening to the healing CD I had made for myself before I went in, doing my breathing exercises several times a day and ensuring I coughed in the correct way, despite how much it hurt to do so. However, another patient who had had the same operation a week earlier and still could not get up commented on how focused I was. Then I contracted a very severe MRSA infection. Fortunately, I was then able to switch my attention to clearing the infection.

Getting through things is about determination. It is also about being able to have the right belief. I never doubted my recovery for a moment. I just focused on asking my mind to tell me everything I needed to know in order to achieve perfect health.

It is incredibly difficult to recover from an illness if you are told you will never recover and you choose to believe it. Have you ever accepted as fact that you will never recover from fibromyalgia/CFS? Resolve today to change this belief. I am testament to the fact this is not the case and that you can recover.

When I contracted MRSA I knew some of my visitors would say, 'Oh! isn't it terrible,' or 'It's awful,' which was the last thing I needed to hear. While others would try to be encouraging by saying, 'Don't be discouraged' or 'Don't be frustrated'. But your unconscious mind doesn't process negation so, of course, I would immediately have taken on these emotions and thought patterns. I could not allow that to happen, so my husband arranged for them not to come until I was in control. Obviously, I would have preferred not to have contracted MRSA, but once I knew I had it, I did not spend even one minute thinking – why me? And I made sure everyone knew I was fine and dealing with it.

I had the great privilege of working for a company founded by the late Thomas Edison, who held a world record of 1,093 patents for inventions such as the light bulb. There were many stories about him and quotes he was renowned for saying that show how much he believed in what he was doing and that he never gave up. These are two of my favourites by Thomas Edison himself:

1. Many of life's failures are people who did not realise how close they were to success when they gave up.

2. It is without exaggeration that I can say I have constructed 3,000 different theories in connection with the electric light, each one of them reasonable and apparently likely to be true. Yet only in two cases did my experiments prove the truth of my theory. I do not regard any of the previous attempts as a failure; they were merely eliminating ways that did not work.

Believe you can manage your condition

It is so much easier to make things happen if you believe strongly that it will. Try the following exercise:

1. Think of something that you strongly believe in. (That the sun will come up tomorrow, for example.)

2. Notice what images, sounds and feelings arise as you think about this belief and how certain you feel about it.

    a) Is the image black-and-white or colour?

    b) Is it still or moving?

c) Is there any sound?

d) Does it have a border?

e) Where is the image positioned in relation to your body (for example, at eye level to the left-hand side about 30 centimetres away)?

f) Is it accompanied by a happy, relaxed feeling?

3. Now think about recovering from fibromyalgia/CFS.

4. Notice any images, sounds and feelings that arise when you focus on this thought and your uncertainty about it.

a) Is the image black-and-white or colour?

b) Is it still or moving?

c) Is there any sound?

d) Does it have a border?

e) Where is the image positioned in relation to your body (for example, directly in front of you at about eye level, with an accompanying emotion that is anxious, worried or nervous)?

5. The images themselves are different, but have you noticed the other differences between the images?

6. The details of the images such as the position of the image, accompanying sounds, etc., are called sub-modalities. Now visualise each sub-modality of your belief about recovering from fibromyalgia/CFS and change them to match those of your positive belief. Do this by imagining each change one by one – move the image, change the sounds, etc.

Once you have completed the exercise:

1. Seek out information about other people, like me, who have recovered or at least improved their lifestyle and enjoyment of life.

2.   Find a trigger event around which to begin to transform your belief, like reading my book.

3.   Enjoy how it feels to have this new belief.

4.   Start by taking steps in line with your new belief about yourself, like doing the exercises in my book.

I can understand if you feel that the sun coming up and your ability to be pain-free are too different, in that you know the sun will come up as a fact and therefore do not regard it as a belief. If this is the case, choose a belief of your own that you cannot prove but instinctively know it is true. For me, this would be that my husband and daughter love me. I cannot prove it and I may not even be able to explain it very well, but it is as true to me as the fact that the sun will rise tomorrow and I don't need evidence.

☺ The first reaction of many of my clients is that they cannot make or conjure images. This is because they are thinking too consciously. Once they relax, they are amazed at the images that they have been creating all the time without even being aware of them.

When I was recovering I knew I needed to be very determined and focused on my recovery. In order to reinforce and energise your belief that you will recover, do the following exercise every day:

Determination visualisation

1.   Imagine yourself fully recovered:

   a)   see what you would see

   b)   hear what you would hear

   c)   notice what you would be doing

   d)   sense how good you would feel

   e)   really imagine it vividly

   f)   ensure the image you have created is motivating, powerful and appealing to you.

I had several really compelling visions of myself being happy, healthy and fit at various times in my future. I was thrilled, as in the months and years that followed, they began to come true, just as I had envisaged.

2. Imagine being fully recovered from fibromyalgia/CFS:

    a) Recall any negative suggestion that anyone gave you about not recovering.

    b) Hear them say, but it in a voice you do not trust or believe – you can make it sound silly and squeaky or like a cartoon character. Choose whatever tone will hold the least power over you.

    c) Promise yourself in a confident and certain tone of voice that you will recover fully.

    d) Remember all the times you got through difficult situations and how at the end of it you were a stronger person as a result of the experience.

3. Next, focus on those times and remember how it felt to be determined enough to get through anything:

    a) see what you saw

    b) hear what you heard

    c) feel what you felt

    d) notice where you had this feeling in your body

    e) give it a colour – one that represents positivity and happiness to you

    f) imagine the colour glowing inside you like a healing light.

4. Promise yourself once again that you will regain good health and get the life you want:

    a) say it with determination

    b) imagine getting through it and recovering

    c) see what you will see

d)   hear what you will hear

e)   feel what you will feel

f)   make the image really compelling

g)   make it into a mini movie in your mind.

Practise this exercise often until you can easily recall your vision and immediately invoke positive feelings of determination. Then any time you feel like giving up trying to recover, replay the movie in your mind and feel the positive feelings that go with it.

Your unconscious works best when it has an image, because this makes it easier to create things. If you were asked to paint a picture of a flower and you had never seen one and so had no concept of what one is like or what a petal is, for example, it would be almost impossible for you to do so. By doing this exercise, you are giving your unconscious mind something to aim for. In the exercise, the image you are creating is your goal and it is a lot easier to get to your destination on your journey if you know what or where it is you are aiming for.

Create a calm environment – de-clutter your life

Throughout this guide you will find many exercises and suggestions to de-clutter and calm your mind. But your environment is also important. The fact is, your sense of calmness and control over your environment is vastly improved by order.

Most adults feel they need to be on top of things to be in control. By maintaining an environment that is ordered, we feel that we have created that order ourselves and the satisfaction can be reassuring.

The stress caused by clutter can be enormous. Being in a cluttered environment increases anxiety about all the things you need to do, as well as making all of the tasks more difficult, thereby increasing stress levels.

☺ Every time you cannot find something, your stress levels can shoot up as you waste valuable time looking

– and then you may start to think it is your 'brain (fibro) fog' that made you lose it.

Stress, in turn, lowers your immunity and resistance, to the degree that your health may suffer even more. Clutter can also affect your self-esteem if you begin to feel like you are missing some basic skill that everyone else appears to have, making you feel bad about yourself. You may even start to feel like you aren't a good parent or a good example to your kids. The truth is, you are not alone – many people have issues dealing with clutter.

Some people believe that clutter drains your energy, which is not good if you are a fibromyalgia/CFS sufferer with limited energy as it is. This concept is based on the understanding that every item in your home has an energy of its own. If items are left unused or uncared for, they become stagnant energy that can actually physically drain you of your energy.

Clutter causes irritability and resentment, which in turn can lead to disagreements within families, especially if people have to deal with other people's clutter. The ability of children to focus may also be affected by clutter. We all know how easily children can be distracted, so it makes sense to give them an environment that is clutter-free. Even people's social life can be affected by clutter, because they may avoid entertaining or having visitors round at home. Or perhaps the energy it would take to find their clothes, etc., for a night out is too overwhelming and so they don't do it at all.

I believe clutter decreases your ability to enjoy life. It causes stress, confusion and an inability to focus, often leading to depression. In my experience, once people start letting go of their clutter, their energy comes back and depression can begin to lift.

It is possible to prove this for yourself. Ensure that just one room is meticulously maintained, with nothing out of place. Keep it like this even if the rest of the house becomes untidy. Try sitting in the tidy room for a while and then move to the untidy part. Then move back. Notice the difference in how relaxed you feel when you return to the tidy room.

☺ I can almost hear you shouting: 'How am I meant to get organised when I'm exhausted!'

Simply choose a small area to start with. If you decide to sort out one drawer, for instance, set a timer for ten minutes and put on some happy music. Completely empty it and give it a quick clean. As you pick up each item, ask yourself: Why am I keeping this? Do the tidying in small bursts, so you don't tire yourself out. Tidy out one thing or space every day according to your energy levels; this activity could even be your exercise for the day.

Once you have decided to let go of belongings and get rid of them, it is crucial to get them out of the house as soon as possible. Give unwanted items to charity, friends, family or recycle them. You could even sell them to bring in some extra cash. As you put things in the bin or charity shop bag, you may feel great, accompanied by a sense of relief, or you may feel guilty that you are wasting money by throwing things away.

You might feel guilty that you are letting go of unwanted presents or baby clothes. I know many people feel it is wrong to discard photos. Or perhaps you feel the moment you get rid of it you will need it. These feelings are perfectly normal, but the rewards of de-cluttering are so great that believe me, it is worth persevering.

Perhaps choose a beautiful box in which to keep sentimental items. If someone gives you an unwanted gift and there is no polite way to refuse, accept gracefully and respect the other person's feelings. Perhaps you could give it to a charity and raise money for a good cause with your donation. If you really feel anxious about letting go of something, store it for six months in the loft or shed. If you still haven't used it after this period then give it away.

I take unwanted items to my local charity shops at least once a month, because I firmly believe that it is far better to have items raising money for good causes than having them cluttering up my home.

☺ In the past my husband has commented that it is mainly his stuff I think of as junk!

It is easy to maintain a tidy home if you operate the 'touch it once' principle – in other words, when you have finished with an item, put it away. It will save you loads of energy because you won't have to tidy up before cleaning as everything is already in its place.

Summary

At this point I feel that I need to mention that I do not think other people need to study the power of the mind to the level I did in order to recover. I did it because I decided I wanted to help other people by becoming a coach and because the subject fascinated me. In fact, I was completely gripped by the topic from day one. Having an additional goal also aided my recovery because it gave me another focus, which meant that I was not just thinking about my illness and obsessing about my recovery.

I have met other people who have been very determined to recover but, unfortunately, their feelings of determination have been marred by desperation and fear of failure. Whereas I felt absolute certainty that I would recover and was filled with joy and excitement at the possibilities for my future.

So before you move on to the next chapter, ensure you have practised the determination visualisation and that you believe you *can* recover. Don't put unnecessary time constraints on yourself and enjoy the journey. For me, this will be a continuous pleasurable, lifelong journey of learning and improving my enjoyment of life.

Key Steps to My Recovery

- Recognise that all information received is being deleted, distorted and generalised.
- Realise that how you experience everything is just your perception.
- Actively notice the good things you have previously deleted from your awareness.
- Accept responsibility for everything in your life.
- Resolve to recover using a powerful visualisation technique.
- De-clutter your environment.

Chapter Four – Exhaustion

Life is either a daring adventure or nothing.

Helen Keller.

Introduction

Exhaustion was one of the most difficult things for me to cope with and I found it incredibly frustrating because prior to developing fibromyalgia/CFS I was an energetic, successful person who could achieve huge amounts every day. I completed a three-year course in just two years while working over seventy hours a week and I still found time to work out at the gym several times a week. Naturally, when I was unable to find the energy to do simple things like housework, walk my daughter to school and on really bad days even wash my own hair, you will understand how I was upset.

> ☺ Although, I now admit that the way I lived my life at top speed probably contributed to my developing fibromyalgia.

The worst part of suffering exhaustion was how irritable it made me feel. I would find myself snapping at those I love the most and would then feel terrible about it afterwards. My husband was always patient but, of course, he could never hope to understand, because one of the things about fibromyalgia/CFS is that you look healthy on the outside. He knows me so well that he could see when I was tired just by looking at my eyes, but even he could not gauge the intensity.

In my opinion, the best way to understand why you are so exhausted is like this: every day we all have a certain amount of energy available to us and if we are using up excessive energy through being stressed or by multitasking, we will soon feel tired out. We all need regular rest periods but, unfortunately, the more we sit around doing nothing, the more lethargic we will feel. So we also need to get moving again – but I know first-hand how hard it is to get started when suffering from this condition.

Focus on the Task in Hand

In today's hectic world many of us have become very skilled at doing two or even three things at once.

☺ Or at least women have.

But seriously, perhaps it is no coincidence that most fibromyalgia (FMS) sufferers are women. Men generally focus on one thing at a time and appear to be unable to think or chat about anything else while doing it, while women are almost always dividing their attention. The problem is that this uses up far more energy, especially if the other thing they are doing while vacuuming, for instance, is worrying!

Think of it like this – you only have so much energy to use each day and if vacuuming takes up one unit and planning what to eat for supper takes one unit, you might expect the equation to look like this: $1 + 1 = 2$ units of energy expended. But if you are doing them both at the same time, it is more likely to look like this: $1 + 1 = 4$. And if the second task is something you are worrying about it is even worse: $1 + 1 = 11$.

So it makes sense to do one thing at a time and difficult as you might find it to believe, you will actually get more done because you will get things done quicker. You can save on energy and time and enjoy tasks far more if you learn to focus 100 per cent on what you are doing. It is not easy after years of multitasking, but it is worth it.

Be persistent and focus fully on at least one task at a time every day for at least five minutes.

Eye of the Storm

For people with fibromyalgia/CFS, one of the most exhausting things is interacting with other people, particularly at social or other events where there are lots of people. I now find it easy to enjoy an event without becoming pulled into the frenzy of activity as everyone else vies for attention. I am not talking about just sitting there zombified in a corner while everyone else has fun – I am talking about observing, listening and calmly contributing to the fun.

If you start off by practising this technique at social events, you will actually find that you enjoy the events more. As you become more skilled, you will be able to use the same technique on occasions that are more difficult.

Several years ago my husband and I were enjoying a holiday with three of our children, when the TV news advised that a hurricane was heading our way. Being the wonderfully protective husband and father that he is, he immediately took steps to have us moved to a safe location, where we awaited the storm.

As the storm moved closer, we all sat in the same room playing a game to distract the children while the storm raged. Appearing to grow in strength each moment, the torrential rain and deafening wind clearly announced the violent storm. Then there was an eerie silence as the wind almost stopped and stillness descended on us – we were in the eye of the storm! The period of calm was short-lived, as the hurricane moved on leaving uprooted trees, upturned cars and damaged buildings in its wake. It is not the hurricane itself that left an impact on me but the calm and tranquillity of the eye of the storm. It was so peaceful amidst the chaos and believe it or not, it is possible to live in the eye of the storm of challenging events.

One thing that will certainly leave you exhausted is a large surge of adrenaline caused by stress and panic. It is not easy to stay calm internally as well as externally. I was an expert at appearing calm and relaxed in the face of a crisis, but inside I was in turmoil. Now, my sense of calmness starts on the inside.

As I explained earlier, it is best to begin practising inner calmness at social events. Imagine you are in a situation where everyone around you is vying for attention, trying to get their opinions across. At such times it can be exceedingly taxing, even triggering a fibro (brain)-fog attack. This leads to frustration and before you know it, you are feeling exhausted.

Thankfully, there is a way you can step back from it all and enjoy the experience by being in the eye of the storm. Here are my tips for being calm in the storm:

1. Breathe deeply.
2. Listen to other people without the intention of putting your opinion across.
3. Let others be right and have the glory.
4. Ask if there is anything you can learn from the way people are behaving.
5. Only speak when you have something that is pleasant, constructive or amusing to say.
6. Use your calming anchor (explained later).

Learning to be Flexible

Trying to stick rigidly to plans is extremely exhausting and usually counterproductive, maybe even resulting in you pushing yourself excessively, making you feel worse. By becoming more flexible you will find that without any effort, wonderful changes happen all by themselves. You will become more relaxed and yet you will actually achieve more, because you will be focusing on results rather than expending energy agonising about the details of how you will achieve them.

If I were a stick of rock, I would have the words 'happiness' and 'gratitude' running through me, but many years ago those words would have been 'anxiety' and 'stress'. Being a perfectionist meant that if I started a project, I finished it – no matter what. This certainly led to my being very successful at whatever I did, but it also meant that I would get very stressed if my plans had to change or things overran. In turn, this would make me feel exhausted.

No matter how well you plan, there are countless times when your plans have to change unexpectedly; for instance, if someone does not do what they said they would or something does not happen as it should. It is understandable that you may become frustrated about it, but these feelings are not helpful to you either emotionally or physically, and can manifest themselves in the form of a flare-up.

Tips to becoming more flexible

Expect a certain percentage of your plans to change, because if you are expecting change it will be less irritating and tiring to sort out when the inevitable happens. Ask yourself:

- What really matters about this situation?
- Am I still able to achieve my desired outcome?
- Can these new circumstances lead to an even better result if I am flexible?
- In what way can I change my desired outcome and still be happy?

Usually, as long as you can achieve the same outcome, the way you achieve it is generally not that important. There is definitely more than one route to happiness.

Challenges

There is no doubt that when you have fibromyalgia/CFS, the strain of dealing with challenges can strip you of the small amount of energy you do have and make symptoms feel much worse. But challenges are a natural part of life and no matter how hard you try, you cannot isolate yourself from obstacles and problems. Although most people think that they will be happy when they have got rid of their problems, true happiness actually comes from changing our relationship to our problems. This means developing the ability to see our challenges as potential for growth.

In the Buddhist tradition it is felt that when life is too easy there are fewer opportunities for genuine growth. Challenges are considered to be so important to a life of growth and peace that a Tibetan prayer actually asks for them: 'Grant that I may be given appropriate difficulties and suffering on this journey so that my heart may be truly awakened'.

Letting Things Wait

Are you the kind of person who obsesses about getting things done in accordance with your imaginary deadlines?

> ☺ I know I was – and still would be if I did not keep myself in check.

The constant battle to manage daily tasks is exhausting enough, without adding self-imposed deadlines. There are always things we have to do by a certain time, like take the children to school, but in all honesty is the world going to collapse if you have not filled the dishwasher first when you could do it when you get back?

> ☺ Confession: this was me – and it was not just about the dishwasher. My house had to look like a show home by 7.30 every morning!

I am not suggesting that you continually leave everything until another time. Just be realistic about the urgency. If you constantly feel as though you are dashing around, it will increase your stress levels and reduce your ability to cope with pain. This only adds to the feelings of exhaustion associated with fibromyalgia/CFS.

> ☺ I will never lose sight of the fact that my health and happiness and that of those I love is the most important thing and that most of the things I have worried about in the past really don't matter. If I remain focused on this and try to be a positive impact on the lives of people I meet in my life on a daily basis, I am able to feel good about my actions.

Managing Your Time Effectively

If you have more things to be done than you have the time or energy for, then managing your time effectively is essential. This is particularly important so that you do not feel stressed at the end of the day about all the things you intended to achieve but have not managed. Worrying about tasks you haven't completed will certainly aggravate the amount of pain you feel and reduce your ability to sleep well. I can achieve a great amount in a short time.

> ☺ This means I have lots of spare time for doing the things I enjoy most.

I find the most efficient way to get things done is to make a list of everything I think I need to do and prioritise them in order of importance. This really helps me to recognise how many things I have on the list that do not really need to be done at all, in which case I can simply cross them off.

> ☺ You might find this difficult at first because you would not have put them on the list if they did not need doing – would you?

The best way to check this is to ask yourself what will happen if this task never gets done. Is there another way to achieve the result you want without doing it? It can be very liberating to realise how much free time you can have by not wasting it engaging in unnecessary tasks. You can then work through the remaining tasks, dealing with each one through to completion; unless of course you are waiting for someone else to come back to you about something. Half doing one task after another is a great time-waster and is a trap many people fall in to, so if possible complete one task before moving on to the next.

Big or Important Events

Many people look forward to big events like weddings and Christmas with a mixture of excitement and dread. Just the worry of whether or not you will be well enough to cope with the event can trigger a flare-up. You have to plan ahead, because there are a thousand things that need to be done and there are all kinds of things that could potentially go wrong. For instance, what if the journey tires you out too much or puts you in too much pain?

When I went to my niece's wedding, because the journey to the church took an hour, I was worried that I would not be able to cope. In the event, my husband took a day off work so we could travel over the day before and we stayed in a hotel opposite the church; even then we had to sneak off in the middle of the day so I could rest.

All too often we take away much of the pleasure of organising an event by worrying about how terrible it will be if the flowers aren't quite right on a wedding day or if the sprouts aren't perfect on Christmas Day. I know that when my symptoms were at their worst, just the thought of trying to organise Christmas was exhausting. One year I was so bad on Christmas Eve that I was unable to help put the children's presents out and I spent Christmas Day lying on the sofa watching them play while my husband did everything else. I found it incredibly distressing not being able to get up and play with them or help with the meal. With this thought in mind, I think it is important to give you some practical tips for surviving big events that you can use in conjunction with the other techniques in this book:

1. Write a list of all the preparation that has to be done in advance of the event.

2. Highlight five or six really important things that if they go well will mean you have a great day, even if other things go wrong.

3. Give yourself time to make decisions calmly and to get the tasks done.

4. Delegate tasks.

5. Take as much pressure off yourself as you can. For example, by shopping online for some of the presents or food. This can be difficult if, like me, you enjoy looking for presents in person, but once you get into it, it is really easy and a lot quicker. It also means you don't waste money on useless impulse buys.

    ☺ Once you have recovered, you will be able to do all kinds of things again without suffering the consequences afterwards.

6. Do whatever it takes so that you can feel relaxed and look forward to the event, even if this means letting go of some of your beliefs about how things should be!

7. Think about what you really want from the day or event and imagine laughing and enjoying yourself.

8. Make sure that all your jobs, or as many as possible, are completed two days beforehand so that you can rest or, better still, book yourself a massage or pamper yourself at home.

9. Accept that events are rarely perfect. Instead, make it as good as you can and enjoy it no matter what small things go wrong.

Understand Others Before Trying to be Understood

The next time someone says something you disagree with, instead of instantly defending your own position, see if you can understand their point of view by asking questions without a hidden agenda of catching them out or proving them wrong.

People often waste hours or even days holding onto their position tightly as if it were a life raft in an ocean of rage. Sadly, this limits opportunities to learn anything new. And for fibromyalgia/CFS sufferers, this surge of negative emotion is likely to cause a flare-up!

Quite simply, if you are arguing with someone, your unconscious mind perceives that you are in some way under threat. It does not realise that someone leaving the top off the toothpaste is not life-threatening when you are shouting about it or putting importance around it. Your unconscious mind just assumes it must be important for you to be reacting the way you are and so initiates the fight or flight response.

Ask yourself how many times you have had a big or long, drawn-out argument in which you have exhausted yourself trying to prove your point, only to realise at the end of it that you are not really sure what the argument was about in the first place. You might be surprised to learn that it is not the person who is right who wins an argument but the one who has the most certainty! So if you have ever walked away from an argument feeling very smug or satisfied because you were right, it is just possible you weren't …

Every time you get upset with another person, remember you are not upset with that individual person – you are upset because they have broken your rules or standards. Next time you are involved in an argument, step back and listen to the other person while asking yourself these questions:

- How could they be right?
- What is more important: my rule or my relationship with this person?

The Old Lady and the Travellers

It was a beautiful day in a land far away as an elderly lady sat resting on the front porch of her cottage that nestled at the edge of a vast river. As she stroked the ginger tom who lay contented on her knee, a traveller came strolling down the road towards her. He hailed the old woman and greeted her warmly. She returned the greeting with a friendly smile.

The traveller explained that he was on his way to a village on the other side of the river and he asked: 'What are the people in the city south of the river like?'

The old maid looked the fellow up and down before asking: 'Where are you from?'

'I hail from Chyrus in the east. I have lived there my entire life,' he replied with a warm smile.

'First, tell me, what are the people of Chyrus like?' she asked.

The happy traveller replied, 'The people of Chyrus are generally well mannered, warm, friendly and caring. It is a good town because the people who live there are good people.'

The old maid smiled. 'My friend, you will find that the people in the city south of the river are very similar to those of Chyrus.'

Happily, the young man took his leave to journey across the river.

The old maid was just about to enter the cottage to prepare her lunch, when a second traveller came by. She greeted the second young man warmly and he also asked what the people in the city south of the river were like. Again, the old woman asked where he was from. Low and behold, the second traveller was also from Chyrus.

But when the old maid asked the fellow what the people of Chyrus were like, he responded: 'Oh! They are mean, selfish and greedy. No one has any time for strangers. It is a terrible place, full of low-life and nastiness. I couldn't wait to get out of there. I have lived there my entire life.'

The wise old woman smiled and sighed as she replied: 'I am sorry to tell you this, young fellow, but you will find the people in the city south of the river are exactly as those of Chyrus.'

Crestfallen, he thanked her for the warning and set off in the opposite direction, telling her he would travel north instead. The wise old dear wished him luck in his search for a town of good people.

Meditation

Many people understand the concept of power-napping, where you take a short nap and wake up feeling refreshed. But when you have fibromyalgia/CFS this just doesn't work. During the day, like many, I generally ended up sleeping for hours and still woke up feeling exhausted.

Meditation is a relaxing activity, so it might sound odd to suggest that you can use it to increase your energy. But in my experience meditation is the best way to get the benefits of napping without actually going to sleep.

I developed a wonderful meditation for myself that I would do three or four times a day. It was only seven minutes long but left me feeling re-energised. I cover meditation in more detail in my chapter on sleep difficulties, and even more in the final chapter – this is just to get you started.

Meditation – step one

1. I chose a simple physical object I could actually hold in my hand to focus on. I selected an orange (fruit), because it reminds me of the power of the sun. Any object will do – it doesn't have to be something simple.

2. I would focus on the orange thinking about the shape, colour and texture, just rolling it around in my hand. I used all of my senses, listening to it, smelling it, touching it with my tongue, etc.

3. When I was able to focus on the orange continuously for two minutes, I knew that I was then ready to focus on myself internally.

Meditation – step two

1. I would take three deep breaths, holding each breath for a moment before making a slight 'harr' sound with each exhalation.

2. Imagining a piece of gold thread holding me up straight towards the sky, I would continue to breathe deeply while repeating the following affirmations:

    a) I am filled with the energy of the sun.

    b) My body is stronger and fitter every day.

    c) I am grateful that I am pain-free.

    d) I appreciate and enjoy the increased energy I am feeling every day.

    e) Thank you for bringing me perfect health.

I would repeat the exercise, starting again at the beginning once I had said all of the affirmations. I would also add other positive affirmations or think about the thread. If other thoughts drifted into my mind I would allow them to float out again. I continued this exercise for five to seven minutes. There are lots of guided meditations available, including mine, but it is possible to develop your own. For further information, please visit:

<http://www.forgetfibromyalgia.com>.

Summary

As I am sure many of you will already have discovered, resting is not effective in managing the level of exhaustion caused by fibromyalgia/CFS. Therefore, a more proactive and whole life approach is required. This is why the information contained within this chapter is intended to help you to manage your time effectively. It is also aimed to reduce the symptoms of fatigue caused by the challenges we face in life through meditation, so that you can learn to relax deeply, perhaps for the first time in many years. This is very much just the starting point in managing your exhaustion and later chapters are packed with information that will help improve your energy levels through a variety of techniques and approaches.

Key Steps to My Recovery

- Let things wait.
- Manage your time effectively.
- Learn to be calm in the eye of the storm.
- Plan sensibly for big events.
- Understand others before trying to be understood.
- Practise meditation.

Chapter Five – Exercise

Take care of your body.
It's the only place you have to live.

Jim Rohn

CAUTION:

Always seek advice from your GP, hospital or a qualified medical professional before undertaking an exercise programme or changing your existing regime.

Introduction

Regardless of my work schedule or other commitments, I still found time to work out at the gym several times a week. So naturally when illness prevented me from doing so, I noticed the negative impact on my body and my general well-being almost immediately.

During the first few years of suffering with fibromyalgia/CFS I tried to walk every day and although this greatly lifted my spirits, I almost always overexerted myself and would spend the afternoon and evening in great pain. This is definitely not recommended.

☺ I think of this as my crash-and-burn stage.

It should be noted that I was physically unable to do household chores like vacuuming carpets at this point.

☺ We replaced as many of the carpets as possible with hardwood flooring and where we were unable to do this, my husband would vacuum for me.

I also had to accept that if I was going to do housework, I could not do the whole house on the same day.

☺ Instead, I would concentrate on one room a day.

This was not easy for me to come to terms with because I have always been very house-proud, but I knew I had to let this go if I was going to recover enough to live a normal life.

☺ It was a real test of my strength of mind not to notice the dust on the mantelpiece.

This section contains mainstream information and guidance widely available regarding fibromyalgia/CFS and exercise, together with details of my own recovery programme. As fatigue is one of the main symptoms of fibromyalgia/CFS, you may feel unable to exercise. However, an exercise programme that is specifically suited to you, which takes into account your current physical condition, can help you to manage your symptoms, as well as improve your overall health.

☺ I believe that becoming increasingly active was fundamental to my recovery.

It is impossible for me to recommend the right exercise programme specifically for your particular condition. The only safe way for you to begin a sensible exercise regime is to speak to a qualified medical practitioner who can recommend a suitable programme.

Your GP, physiotherapist (health-care professional trained in using physical techniques to promote healing) or consultant can help you design a personal exercise programme, which is likely to involve a range of:

- moderately intense aerobic exercises
- strengthening exercises

Aerobic exercises

Aerobic activities are basically any kind of rhythmic, moderate-intensity exercises that use the large muscles in your legs and buttocks. The workout should raise your heart rate, make you breathe slightly harder and make you feel warmer. A good way to confirm if you are working at a moderately intense level is that you should still be able to talk, but not sing the words to a song – your current level of fitness and health are taken into consideration. There are some gentle aerobic classes available at health clubs. Most clubs have classes for all ages and levels of fitness – it is not all about pushing yourself to the limits. Examples of aerobic exercise include:

- walking
- cycling
- swimming in warm water.

A number of studies have found that aerobic exercises may relieve pain. Because I was sensible and increased my exercise levels gradually without overexerting myself (as I had in the past), exercise was definitely beneficial by helping to reduce my fibromyalgia/CFS pain, increasing my energy levels and improving my general sense of well-being.

> ☺ Walking with my dogs was great for me. We had two Teacup Yorkshire terriers – a breed specially chosen by my husband, who researched how much exercise each breed required and came to the conclusion they were practically stuffed! As it turned out, they were perfect; they were equally happy to go on long or short walks or just as content to curl up in front of the fire.

Strengthening exercises

These exercises focus on strength training, such as weightlifting, and they need to be planned as part of a personalised exercise programme. It is vital that you are shown how to do them correctly; otherwise, they can make muscle stiffness and soreness worse. Even healthy people suffer from muscle soreness if they do not follow a sensible plan or do an exercise in the wrong way. And for fibromyalgia/CFS sufferers, it is vital to seek professional advice.

Studies show that strengthening exercises may improve:

- muscle strength
- physical disability
- depression
- quality of life.

My personal plan included a variety of gentle activities, combining both aerobic and muscle-strengthening exercises. Exercise was beneficial in that:

- my mood improved greatly
- I could concentrate better
- I had more energy
- I had less muscle stiffness
- I slept better.

In recent years I have discovered the many advantages of yoga, but for me this was a revelation – the weekly sessions are of great benefit to both my mind and my body.

Yoga

Yoga originated in India about 5,000 years ago. It focuses on strength, balance, breathing and flexibility, and is used to boost mental and physical wellness. It comprises a series of movements called postures. Yoga classes can be found in most health clubs, leisure centres, and even hospitals and surgeries. Yoga is generally regarded as a safe and effective form of exercise. Evidence also suggests that regular yoga is beneficial for relieving aches and pains, including lower back pain.

Pacing yourself

☺ This involves balancing periods of activity with periods of rest and not overdoing it. If you are one of the sufferers of fibromyalgia/CFS who constantly push yourself and then spend days paying for it – like I did for a while – it could slow down your progress in the long run. Over time, you can gradually increase your levels of activity, while making sure that they are balanced with rest.

Patients with pain and fatigue understandably decrease their activity levels, thereby gradually becoming less fit, which in turn increases these symptoms. Exercise can help prevent this downward spiral. Since my condition was very severe it was important that I started at a very low level of exercise and increased gradually, beginning with gentle exercise for three minutes, three times per day.

Initially, this involved just moving around at home to a song that evoked feelings of happiness. Crazy as this might sound, it always cheered me up. If my daughter was at home I would dance with her, which she loved because it made her laugh. Some days, if I felt like I needed fresh air, I would dance in my garden. I progressed to two songs over a period of two weeks.

☺ Fortunately, our garden was not overlooked by neighbours.

Then I began walking, limiting myself to ten minutes three times a day, gradually building this up to thirty minutes twice a day. Once I was able to do thirty minutes of exercise at this level without causing an adverse reaction, I increased the intensity by walking faster and by taking up swimming. At first I thought I would look silly going to the swimming baths and hardly doing any swimming. I was also concerned that my arms would ache, as walking would not have strengthened them sufficiently to be able to swim. But I soon realised that no one was taking any notice of me and began to enjoy the sensation of being supported by the water. Instead, I focused on improving my stroke; if I could only do a few lengths, I was happy with that.

> ☺ I like the saying: 'You would not worry so much about what people think of you if you realised how little they do'.

Warming-up and cooling-down stretches are essential part of any exercise regime and even more so for fibromyalgia/CFS sufferers. I always take time to stretch both before and after exercising.

Important points

While walking I would ensure that my mind was not focused on any discomfort or on how tired I felt at the start of the walk. This was because I knew that if I walked with the correct mindset, I would feel better when I got back.

I would:

1. Focus on enjoying the surrounding countryside.
2. List all the things in my life that I was grateful for.
3. Listen to music.
4. Repeat affirmations related to wellness:

    a) I am feeling fitter and stronger every day.
    b) I am grateful that I am not in pain.
    c) It feels good to be outside in the fresh air.
    d) It is good to know that walking is helping my body to grow strong again.

Do not exercise near bedtime (at least three hours beforehand) as this can make it more difficult for you to sleep. This subject will be covered in the chapter on sleep difficulties.

Posture

It is important to stand as straight as you can and to keep your head up, with your shoulders back. Holding your head up allows you to take in the outside world, rather than looking inward and focusing on any feelings.

There were times when I could only walk if I used my hiking stick and even though this might mean that I was leaning forward slightly, I still kept my head up. I used a hiking stick instead of a walking stick because it made me feel as though I looked less incapacitated by my condition. There was the odd day when it felt impossible to walk any distance other than around the house. On these days I wore a pedometer and set myself a target of walking 1,000 steps before the end of the day, gradually building this up to 5,000. Occasionally even this was impossible, but the important thing was that I stayed positive, determined and motivated that the following day I would be able to walk my route.

It was not until after my recovery from other illnesses that I was significantly able to increase my exercise levels; though, I still did my exercise routine once I came out of hospital. Because of my wound I was told that I should aim to be able to lift my legs up to about 15 centimetres whilst lying down after a period of six months. In fact, I was able to do significantly better than that. Again, I believe this was because I was sensible but persistent. By this time I was feeling really well and I knew it was time for me to join a gym again.

I began with a very gentle toning programme alongside an aerobic programme, both for thirty minutes, that I would do on alternate days. Generally, I prefer to exercise daily where possible. I now work out five or six times a week. Either at the gym or home, I do a combination cardiovascular and strengthening exercises, and yoga.

☺ I also love to go walking and regularly walk 12 or 13 miles with my friend or my husband – and sometimes much further if I can persuade them. On a day when I am doing a long walk, I don't do any additional exercise that day.

If my schedule prevents me from exercising for a few days I can really tell the difference – not only in my physical condition, but also emotionally.

> ☺ I know that exercise keeps me physically fit and emotionally balanced – and I love it!

But I am not fanatical about it. If there is a day I don't feel like exercising, I regard this as a signal from my body that it is not right for me to exercise that day. Instead, I give myself the day off and certainly do not feel guilty about it. Exercise is part of my life and I intend it to remain that way forever, so it is important that I do not allow it to become an obligation or a chore.

I realise that for some of you exercise in the way I do it is never going to be something you enjoy. If this is the case, why not find a way of exercising that is not really exercise at all. There are many ways to do this, like joining a dance class, playing with children or grandchildren and gardening – find something that works best for you and gives you pleasure as well as exercise.

> ☺ If I had thought about it at the time I would definitely have invested in one of those great big trampolines – for my daughter, of course!

Fresh Air

Our bodies are made up of trillions of cells and each of those tiny cells need a constant supply of oxygen in order to survive. After we take in air through our lungs, our red blood cells pick up the oxygen and carry it to the rest of the cells in our bodies. For cells to be healthy they require sufficient oxygen and healthy cells mean a healthy body.

Energy is made from the oxygen we breathe and the food we eat. Most of us in the Western World are getting enough food; in fact, many of us get too much. But are we getting enough oxygen?

If you are stressed or anxious, you may be breathing high in your chest. This means you will not be using your full lung capacity and therefore you will not be taking in as much oxygen as you could be. Practising breathing so that your belly moves will help you to use all of your lung capacity.

> ☺ Having had a malignant melanoma I am certainly no lover of the sun; in fact, even before I never was. Maybe that was my unconscious mind trying to warn me …!

I do realise, however, that a steady supply of fresh air is very important. Fresh air is comprised of a combination of a number of different gases – oxygen and nitrogen being the most abundant ones. If you are always taking in old, stale air you are depriving your cells, including your brain, of one of the most basic human needs. This is harmful to your overall health and well-being.

When you are suffering from fibromyalgia/CFS, your mobility may be impaired and getting outside can be difficult. If it is cold outside the temptation is to keep the windows and doors closed. Unfortunately, this means the oxygen content and quality of the air will go down as you, and whoever else happens to be in the room, breathe out carbon dioxide and other wastes or toxins that are the by-products of metabolism. The metabolism is the set of chemical reactions that happen in living organisms to maintain life. It is therefore vital either to open the windows or go outside, so you are not breathing the same stale air over and over again.

> ☺ I always tried to get outside even for a short while as soon as I could after getting up, because I knew it was guaranteed to make me feel energised.

Summary

Exercise should always be carried out sensibly. Whenever possible, choose an exercise you enjoy, even if you might not consider it exercising. If you are more active and it is helping you to relax, the chances are that you are on the right track. I exercise because I recognise the positive effects on my body and well-being. This means exercising an appropriate amount, whilst ensuring that it is not aggravating or worsening a condition or injury. There are lots of ways to exercise, many of which are not regarded as exercise in the true sense of the word but can be a great deal of fun.

When I began exercising again I listened to my body and measured the effects of exercise. I found that by using a process of test and measure, I was able to work out what would give me more energy and what would exhaust me. Then I gradually increased the amount I did each day, still testing and measuring the effects.

By maintaining a strong, healthy body that is the correct weight for your height age and sex, you are not putting any additional strain on your joints, bones, muscles and tendons. It also helps you to feel good both emotionally and physically. Engage in different forms of exercise, taking things slowly and gently if you need to. It is possible that as well as reducing your pain, it may open up new avenues of enjoyment and relaxation.

Because I knew that I would have less energy around my menstrual period, I took this into account when scheduling my programme. It was around this time of the month that I would focus on walking or swimming rather than toning or more energetic cardio routines. Frequent rest periods were essential, but by using the rest periods to indulge in one of my hobbies or by practising meditation I found that I did not have the overwhelming loss of energy I had previously suffered. I have listed the main elements of my plan here for you:

Key Steps to My Recovery

- Exercise gently for a few minutes several times a day.
- Combine exercise with periods of rest.
- Avoid overexertion.
- Increase exercise gradually but consistently.
- Always stretch muscles before and after exercise.
- Exercise to music that invokes happy thoughts.
- Focus on positive thoughts while walking.

- Never allow the bad days to make you feel it is pointless.

- Get a good supply of fresh air.

- Make allowances for your menstrual period.

PLEASE REMEMBER:

The information provided throughout this section is mainstream and widely available. It is not intended to be a substitute for medical advice.

Only you know your own body and your unique symptoms. This is not an instruction manual. You should always consult your doctor or health-care professional who is treating you before embarking upon a course of exercise.

Chapter Six – Sleep Difficulties

You're the happiest while you're making the greatest contribution.

Robert F. Kennedy

Introduction

I am not a sleep specialist. Therefore, the information I have shared with you regarding the stages of sleep, etc., is basic information, which is generally available. My aim in learning about sleep was not to become an expert on the science of sleep but to have an overall understanding of the process and its importance so I could focus my attention on how to achieve a great night's sleep.

I do not feel it is necessary for you to have a deep understanding of the sleep process, as I am certain the way a lack of restful sleep affects you has already convinced you of its importance. However, I suggest you take a few minutes to read this chapter, where we also focus on how you can get better sleep.

General Information About Sleep

Difficulty sleeping and fibromyalgia/CFS go hand in hand. It has been estimated that up to 80 per cent of people with fibromyalgia/CFS experience some type of disordered sleep and feel tired, drained and physically incapable of dealing with the stresses associated with their condition. Sleep helps to organise memories, support learning and improve concentration. Proper sleep, especially sleep where you are actively dreaming (REM sleep), may regulate mood as well.

Definition and Causes of Insomnia

Insomnia is generally defined as an individual's inability to sleep. It is often thought of as a symptom that can accompany several medical and psychiatric disorders. Insomnia is characterised by a persistent difficulty in falling asleep and staying asleep, waking too early or where sleep is not restful. Typically, the sufferer will experience difficulties or impairment while awake, also feeling tired, irritable and unable to concentrate the next day.

Insomnia or sleeplessness is not the same as sleep deprivation, where sleep is curtailed as a result of limited opportunity for sleep, such as a nursing a baby or a sick relative, or an inability to sleep owing to excessive noise. Insomnia is classed in two categories:

1   Acute or short-term insomnia lasts for between one and four weeks.

2   Chronic or long-term insomnia lasts for more than four weeks.

Insomnia can be grouped into primary and secondary (comorbid) insomnia. Primary insomnia may also be referred to as an insomnia syndrome. It is a disorder in its own right and often has no obvious cause but may arise from behavioural factors, such as negative conditioning or physiological issues, including hyper-arousal (flight or fight response), which will be covered later. In contrast, secondary insomnia arises from other conditions, including:

1.   Environmental factors: such as an uncomfortable bed, noise, or being too hot or cold.

2.   Shift work: changes in shift patterns and corresponding changes in sleep/wake schedules.

3.   Jet lag: a temporary condition that can cause disturbed sleep patterns and fatigue following air travel across a number of time zones.

4. Lifestyle: eating too late at night, alcohol consumption, nicotine, drugs.

5. Substance use: including prescribed medicines. If you believe you may be suffering from the side effects of any medication, you should consult your GP or medical provider.

6. Psychological: anxiety, depression and grief.

7. Medical: for example, chronic pain caused by various conditions such as fibromyalgia (FMS), osteoarthritis, severe headaches, rheumatoid arthritis.

8. Neurological disorders: including Parkinson's disease, Tourette's syndrome and epilepsy.

9. Sleep disorders: including sleep apnoea syndrome and restless legs syndrome.

Why Sleep is so Important

It is not fully understood why we need to sleep, so perhaps its importance is best explained by understanding the effects of a lack of good, quality sleep. Surveys have reported that many people sleep less than six hours a night and that up to a third of people in the UK have reported having sleep difficulties at some point in their lives. Although it is believed to be more prevalent in women and to increase with age.

Whilst having the occasional disturbed night or bout of sleepless nights may be irritating, a short period of insomnia is generally something your body can cope with and is therefore no cause for concern. However, chronic sleep issues are a very different matter. It is my belief that lack of restful sleep plays a significant part in fibromyalgia/CFS. It is accepted that lack of sleep may contribute to a number of health problems, including:

1. Concentration, Memories and Learning

Sleep helps to consolidate memories, improve concentration and the ability to learn. Sleep deprivation contributes to a greater tendency to fall asleep during the day. Reduced concentration and tiredness may cause falls, mistakes and accidents. Sleep deprivation also affects motor skills and decision-making, to the degree that it can be similar to that of driving whilst drunk if seriously sleep deprived. For me this was a major problem and I even had to stop driving altogether for a while.

2. Cardiovascular Health

Cardiovascular disease increases the chance of having a sleep disorder. Conversely, sleep disorders increase the chance of having cardiovascular disease. Serious sleep disorders have been linked to hypertension, increased stress, hormone levels and an irregular heartbeat.

3. Immune System

Individuals who are continually rushing around are susceptible to viruses the minute they stop or wind down for a holiday or a break. Many people find they come down with a cold having become exhausted after a stressful event or a big project at work that has adversely affected their sleep. Sleep is essential for the immune system. Without adequate sleep, the immune system becomes weak and the body more vulnerable to infection and disease.

Sleep deprivation alters immune function, including the activity of the body's killer cells, which keep the invaders at bay while the rest of the immune system prepares to fight infection. Unlike our other immune cells, they are always at the ready and have the innate ability to recognise viruses and tumour cells immediately, while other immune cells take two to three days to begin their processes.

4. Nervous System

Neurons are the highways of the nervous system that carry out both voluntary commands, like your moving limbs, and essential involuntary commands, like breathing and digestive processes. Sleep is also a time of rest and repair, so you don't have to be a neuroscientist to recognise that a long-term lack of quality sleep is not good for your nervous system.

5. Mood and Emotions

Proper sleep, especially sleep where you are actively dreaming (REM sleep), may regulate mood as well as emotions. Lack of sleep can make even the most easy-going people irritable and cranky, affecting social interaction.

6. Metabolism and Weight

Severe sleep deprivation may cause weight gain by affecting the levels of hormones that control our appetite and also the way we process and store carbohydrates.

7. Hormone Release

Many hormones – substances produced to trigger, stimulate or regulate particular body functions into action – are timed to release during sleep or right before sleep. Growth hormones, for example, are released during sleep – vital not only to growing children, but also for restorative processes like muscle repair.

How Much Sleep is Enough?

All of us need sleep. We sleep to rest our minds and bodies and to restore our energy for the following day, but how much do we need? There have been several famous, successful people who are reported to function incredibly well with very little sleep. There are varying reports that suggest that the artist Leonardo da Vinci was known to sleep one and a half hours a day by sleeping for fifteen minutes every four hours. What effect this had on him we will never know. And we are told that Margaret Thatcher, Florence Nightingale and Napoleon only needed four hours a night.

In reality, there are always exceptions to every rule and it may be possible to train ourselves to function well on less than average sleep. But most of us need a good night's sleep of between seven and eight hours a night in order to wake up feeling refreshed and ready to perform at our best during the day ahead. We all feel sleepy at one time or another. Simply staying up late to watch a film or having a night out can result in feeling tired the next day. While most of us can push through this feeling, if the shortage of sleep continues over a period of time, we can build up a large sleep deficit. This takes its toll on our physical and emotional health, and can result in symptoms similar to those of fibromyalgia/CFS.

How Do Our Bodies Know When it is Time to Sleep?

During the 24-hour cycle of each day, our body and brain alternate between states of high activity during the waking day, and rest and repair during night-time sleep. We all have an internal circadian body clock that provides cues and regulates when it is time to sleep and time to wake. This clock is sensitive to light and time of day, so it is important to have a quiet, dark place in which to sleep in addition to a good bedtime routine.

A chemical messenger called adenosine builds up during the day as our bodies use up our energy reserves. As the levels of adenosine in the brain increase, the sleepier we will feel and combined with the circadian clock, it promotes sleep. Some people believe that it is the build-up of adenosine at the wrong time that causes the extreme fatigue associated with fibromyalgia/CFS – I do not know if this is correct, but once I was getting restful sleep, my fatigue reduced significantly.

The Sleep Cycles

> A ruffled mind makes a restless pillow.
> Charlotte Brontë

There are two main types of sleep. REM (rapid eye movement) sleep is when most active dreaming takes place. It is characterised by the eyes moving back and forth, which is why it is called REM sleep. Non-REM (NREM) sleep consists of varying stages of light and deep sleep. Each sleep stage is important for overall quality of sleep, but deep sleep and REM sleep are especially vital.

For most adults, seven to eight hours appears to be the optimum amount of sleep required. During sleep, the body goes through several stages in a cyclic fashion throughout the night, moving back and forth between deep, restorative sleep and more alert stages and dreaming. As the night progresses we spend more time in longer stages of dreaming (REM sleep), alternated with lighter sleep (stage two – NREM sleep).

REM Sleep (Dream Sleep)

At about seventy to ninety minutes into our sleep cycle we enter REM sleep. We usually have three to five REM episodes per night. This stage is essential to our minds for processing emotions, retaining memories and relieving stress. Breathing is rapid, irregular and shallow, blood pressure rises and the heart rate increases. Most dreaming remains a mystery, but one theory is that dreams may be the brain's way of processing random fragments of information received during the day. If REM sleep is disrupted one night, the body will go through more REM the next night to catch up on this sleep stage.

The Stages of Non-REM Sleep

As explained, NREM sleep is made up of varying levels, from light sleep through to very deep sleep. There are four stages:

1. Stage one (drowsiness) – this is the beginning of the sleep cycle and it is a relatively light stage of sleep, lasting around five to ten minutes. It can be considered to be a transition period between wakefulness and sleep, where the muscles are active and the eyes roll slowly, opening and closing moderately. If you are woken up during this stage, you might believe that you weren't asleep.

2. Stage two (light sleep) – this stage generally lasts for approximately twenty minutes, during which the body temperature decreases and the heart rate slows. The brain begins to produce bursts of rapid, rhythmic brain wave activity and it is more difficult to wake from this stage.

3. Stage three (deep sleep) – transition stage between light sleep and very deep sleep, during which slower brain waves begin to emerge.

4. Stage four (deep sleep) – lasting for approximately thirty minutes, bed-wetting and sleepwalking are most likely to occur at the end of this sleep stage, as it is a very deep stage of sleep from which it is difficult to be

aroused. If your alarm clock wakes you during this stage of sleep, it is highly likely that you will feel very groggy.

It is worth noting that The American Academy of Sleep Medicine no longer designates a stage four, which was once considered the deepest sleep stage. So stage three, previously thought to be a transition to deep sleep, now includes both three and four.

My Sleep Problems

I would get into bed feeling exhausted and as though I could not stay awake a moment longer. Only to find that the minute I lay down I was so uncomfortable from the pain in my neck, muscles and other tender points that there was no position I could lie in that would allow me to fall asleep. Despite being so tired, I would then start going over things in my mind. I would worry about all the things I was not able to do, about how I would cope with things that were coming up and generally about anything and everything in my life.

Eventually I would fall into a light sleep, waking often to try to reposition my body, particularly my neck. The difficulty being that my neck felt better if I lay on my back, but the tender points on my shoulder blades were too painful when they made contact with the mattress. But I also had a tender point on each hip, so lying on my side was equally uncomfortable. Every time I woke up I would need to go to the toilet to urinate, which some nights was seven or eight times. When I got back into bed I would have the same problems drifting back off.

Almost every morning I would wake up feeling unrested. Prior to fibromyalgia/CFS I had always awoken alert and ready for the day, and never had any trouble getting up. Yet, my condition left me feeling like there was no way I could even get out of bed.

Five-Step Formula to Better Sleep

1. Appreciate your day – relax

If you are lying there feeling frustrated thinking about all the things that are wrong in your life, or anxious and stressed, worrying about all the things that could go wrong in the future, it is very difficult to fall into a deep, peaceful sleep. There are three ways that I recommend you use to put yourself in a good mood for sleep:

a.   Deal with the day's challenges

Quickly jot down any concerns or worries you have that day. Take no more than five minutes to do this. Resolve to work on a solution to the problem the next day. Now, instead of lying awake overanalysing every aspect of a problem, challenge or difficult situation, I often forget about the dilemma, confident that within an hour or so of waking up I will have the solution. This is because the unconscious mind has the ability to help you process solutions while you are asleep.

b.   Spend fifteen minutes making a list of all the things in your life that you are grateful for

Whenever I first ask clients to do this, often their first reaction is to feel that they don't have much to be grateful for. I think the smallest list I have seen had three things on it. But once we explore this more deeply their lists quickly expand.

There are so many things people can be grateful for, even when they are feeling ill or facing challenges in life. To help my clients expand their list, I ask them to think about the following:

- things in nature they love
- things they can still do with their bodies like see and hear
- skills and talents they have
- wonderful experiences from their past
- family and friends
- hobbies and pastimes that give them pleasure
- job or career

- TV shows that they enjoy watching

- the pleasure they get from a pet.

Once we have covered these they are usually on a roll and can find many more things.

When you are writing your list, it is important that you don't just write things down without thinking about the pleasure they bring you. You should actually experience the feeling or emotion of being grateful for the things on your list.

☺ My gratitude list has several hundred things on it and it is still growing!

c. **Listen to a pre-recorded relaxation session**

Some people find it much easier to be guided into relaxation. When they try to relax alone they actually become too focused on trying to quieten their mind, which is extremely difficult. If someone else guides them, they can focus on their words instead. This way, they will generally find that they can relax quicker and more deeply. Alternatively, listening to a relaxation CD that is made up of soothing sounds or music can be equally effective, especially when it is tailored to their condition.

If you want to try using my personal meditation, please visit: <http://www.forgetfibromyalgia.com>.

In summary, if you brood about your day or worry about the future, you are making it very difficult for your body to relax and drift into sleep. So my strategy for a good night's sleep focuses on ensuring that you are in the best possible mindset for sleep.

The sleep switch is designed to occupy the mind so that it is difficult to focus on negative thoughts. It also provides a powerful anchor for sleep. As you are climbing into bed, tell yourself that resting with your eyes closed is good for your body and think about all the things you have put on your gratitude list. This will calm your mind and remove any anxious feelings around sleep.

2. My sleep switch (anchor)

The aim of this anchor is for the brain to associate a poem, rhyme or prayer with sleep:

a) Choose a poem, rhyme or prayer that you like. Make sure it is one that is neutral with no memories attached or one that stimulates pleasant and peaceful thoughts.

b) Once you get into bed, begin to recite whatever it is that you have chosen in your head.

c) Repeat it over and over until you fall asleep.

d) If other thoughts or worries come into your head, push them out and start at the *beginning*.

e) If you lose your place, start at the *beginning*.

f) Concentrate on the words so that your mind is focused on whatever it is you have chosen to recite and nothing else.

g) You will need to be very dedicated at repeating this exercise every night, and every single time you wake up during the night, until you drift off to sleep.

h) In the beginning you may need to repeat the recitation many times before you fall asleep.

i) The more you persevere, the quicker your brain will associate the verse with sleep and the faster the results will be.

> NOTE: Your mind will wander, because that is what minds do. Do not become frustrated, because no matter how many times you have to start again, it will not affect the effectiveness of your sleep anchor.

As your switch becomes more effective, you will find that you begin to fall asleep before the end of the verse.

☺ Within just three weeks my sleep switch was surprisingly effective and even after all these years, I cannot say my chosen verse in my head without falling asleep. In fact, I never even get to the end of the verse before I am asleep.

What is a sleep switch?

A sleep switch is actually what is more commonly known as an anchor. Russian physiologist, psychologist and physician Pavlov is widely known for first describing the phenomenon of classical conditioning (anchoring). In the 1890s, Pavlov was investigating the gastric function of dogs, when he noticed that dogs tended to salivate before anything was actually delivered to their mouths and so he set out to investigate further. As a result of carrying out a long series of experiments, he discovered 'conditional reflexes' – like salivation – that only occurred conditionally upon specific previous experiences of the animal.

Unconscious anchors

Anchors are stimuli that call forth thoughts or emotions, and then corresponding actions. In fact, we are constantly affected by and respond to these automatic unconscious anchors, often without realising why our mood has changed or why we have taken a particular action. This is because the anchors have been built up over time. In fact, our responses are so automatic we are almost on autopilot.

Unconscious anchors can be found in many forms. For example, if you have a habit of squeezing your little finger when stressed and then you repeat this action when you are relaxed, it will stimulate your stress response. In addition to affecting your mood, they might produce an automatic involuntary reaction or memory, like answering the phone or stopping as traffic lights turn red. So a certain smell like candyfloss or bacon may take you back to your childhood and a song may remind you of a certain person or holiday. I have become so used to exercising to certain songs that as soon as I hear them, I feel energised.

The first time I heard about an unconscious anchor was at the pain clinic, when the clinical psychologist told us about how he was always getting up late for lectures when he was at university and how he got into the habit of brushing his teeth whilst going to the toilet. Brushing his teeth still stimulated the urge to urinate twenty years later!

3. A bedtime routine

It is vitally important to establish a good bedtime routine:

a) Ensure your bedroom is quiet, dark and a comfortable temperature.

b) Stick to a regular bed/sleep schedule. Support your biological clock by going to bed and getting up at the same time every day, including weekends. Get up at your usual time in the morning even if you are tired. This will help you to get back into a regular sleep rhythm. It is very difficult when you are feeling exhausted, but I found that once I started moving around, particularly if I went for a short walk in the fresh air, I would feel more alert. It also helped maintain a regular sleep rhythm.

c) Avoid naps – napping during the day can make it more difficult to sleep at night. If you feel like you have to take a nap, limit it to thirty minutes before 3.00 p.m. and where possible, do some meditation instead of napping.

d) Avoid stimulating activity and stressful situations before bedtime. This includes big discussions or arguments, vigorous exercise, watching the TV and playing on the computer or video games. I would turn off all electronic appliances at least fifteen minutes before going to bed, get ready for bed by brushing my teeth, etc., and then do something relaxing such as reading, drinking a warm drink, taking a bath or listening to soothing music or a hypnosis CD.

e) Although this was not an issue for me and it did not require a change in my behaviour, I believe that in order to obtain a good night's sleep you should restrict your alcohol, caffeine and nicotine intake; perhaps stop drinking caffeinated beverages at least six hours before bed.

Although alcohol can make you feel sleepy, it interferes with the quality of your sleep. As nicotine is a stimulant, consider quitting smoking or avoid it at night.

f)   Train your body to associate bed with sleep and nothing else – especially not frustration and anxiety. Use the bedroom only for sleeping and intercourse. Don't work, read, watch TV or use your computer in the bedroom. The aim is to associate the bedroom with sleep alone, so that your brain and body get a strong signal that it is time to sleep when you get into bed.

g)   In order to practise abdominal breathing, breathe deeply by involving not only the chest, but also the lower back, rib cage and belly. This can actually help the part of our nervous system that controls relaxation. When I got into bed I would close my eyes and take deep, slow breaths, making each breath even deeper than the last. I would breathe in through my nose and out through my mouth, ensuring each exhalation lasted a little longer than each inhalation. At the same time I would recite my chosen verse – otherwise known as a sleep switch.

4. Awakening with natural light

For me, the worst part of waking up was being jolted wide awake by a blaring alarm clock. Not exactly the best way to start the day! I prefer to use natural light whenever possible to wake up. I find this technique to be a far gentler way to start my day and I feel more alert when I use this method. In fact, my body is so attuned to waking up when I need to that I don't like to set an alarm, even if I have an appointment or a plane to catch, and will only do so when absolutely necessary.

Waking naturally is proven to be the most enjoyable way to start the day, by relying on the gradual increase of natural daylight. However, if you have heavy blackout curtains it is difficult for the light to get in. Also, depending on the time you get up and where you live, there may not be any natural daylight at the time you want to get up.

Nevertheless, there are natural-light alarm clocks available on the market that are designed to wake you up using a soothing, progressively lightening emulator of daylight. It starts dull and gradually brightens so that it feels like you are experiencing the natural sunrise and gradual lightening of the sky. This makes it far easier and more enjoyable for you to wake up, as your body is designed to flow with the natural rhythms of the day. By emulating the sunrise, the natural-light alarm clock works with your body's natural rhythms to wake you up gently.

> ☺ It was not necessary for me to invest in one of these because my lovely husband opened the curtains at six o'clock in the morning when he left for work so that I could wake up gradually. I found this a far nicer way to wake up.

5. Meditation – Step Three

Meditation is a proven alternative therapy that can be broadly classified under mind–body medicine. It is a safe and simple way to balance a person's physical, emotional and mental state, and can benefit anyone.

The value of meditation to promote healing has been known and practised for thousands of years, and is rooted in the traditions of the world's great religions. In fact, practically all religious groups practise meditation in one form or another.

Benefits of meditation

When you are suffering from fibromyalgia/CFS it can drain your energy. In fact, it can be exhausting trying to live a normal life while coping with pain. Meditation is effective in reducing pain and increasing energy, so it has double benefits.

We all need to take quiet time for ourselves and put ourselves in an appropriate state to listen to what our bodies are telling us they need. If we are constantly in a state of anxiety, stress or depression, our bodies will find away to get our attention in a variety of other ways. This might be through illness, discomfort or sudden emotional outbursts; mine certainly did just that. I am now very in tune with my body and this has been a vital element in ensuring that I remain symptom-free. As I practised I found these brief moments of calm became very precious to me and I now believe they are ultimately essential to my leading a happy, healthy life.

Our daily lives are often so hectic that we rarely get the opportunity to focus on just nourishing our inner selves. I had become an expert at ignoring the inner needs and emotions that we all have. Thankfully, I eventually realised it was time to acknowledge those feelings and allow my higher self to bring me the answers I needed for greater happiness and wellness. You can, too – all you have to do is listen.

☺ Give it a go! You have absolutely nothing to lose and only health, energy and happiness to gain!

As I have explained earlier, we all have our own unique circadian rhythms, which means that during the day (every sixty to ninety minutes) our energy levels take a natural dip and we feel tired. Most people ignore these signals from their body and press on with their day, overriding the natural impulse to rest.

If you have fibromyalgia (FMS) or CFS I guess that you, like me, find these dips in energy so overwhelming that you fall asleep. The problem for me was that I rarely felt any better when I woke up: indeed, often I would feel worse.

How to begin meditating

There are many ways of meditating. Everyone can do it because there is no right or wrong way. The important thing to begin with is getting started by taking quiet time for yourself. In order to relax fully, make sure you will not be disturbed. Take the telephone off the hook and switch off any mobiles or alarms. My easy meditation only takes seven minutes, so other people can wait. Remember, this is about you and gaining a pain-free existence, in addition to achieving overall wellness. If finding the time is difficult, think about the last time you spent thirty minutes watching a soap, sit-com or reality TV show and resolve in future to do a meditation instead. Meditating will help you to relax far more than sitting in front of the TV.

☺ I am sure you have heard about people who meditate for an hour or two, but in my experience that will not be necessary for you to begin to feel the benefits of meditation. And let's be honest – most of us would be unable to fit that into our day on a regular basis. Experiment with what works best for you, perhaps doing short meditations with a long session once a week.

You can start with just two minutes and progress to longer periods if you wish. I found short, twice-daily meditations were most effective, but you will soon work out what feels right and works best for you.

1.   Sit in a well-supported chair. The most important thing is to be comfortable so you can relax.

2.   Make sure that your feet touch the ground and are flat on the floor.

3.   Allow your mind to quieten its thoughts and let the body completely relax. There are many ways to quieten your mind and body, such as focusing on a simple object, as in Meditation – step one (see chapter on exhaustion). Listed below is another method that I enjoy:

a)   Focus on your breathing.

b)   Slowing the pace of your breathing, notice the temperature of the breath entering your nostrils.

c)   Inhale deeply, hold for three seconds and then exhale slowly. It is important to breathe through the nose as the body tends to breathe more rapidly through the mouth when highly active or in fight or flight mode. If you are breathing steadily through the nose you will achieve the reverse effect of that pattern.

d)   Continue breathing steadily while counting down slowly from ten to one.

e)   Next, become aware of your feet on the floor and acknowledge that you are rooted to the power of the earth, while continuing to breathe steadily.

f) Visualise yourself walking safely down a very long, beautiful, ornate staircase, getting more relaxed as you take each step, going further and further down. Or perhaps you could visualise yourself strolling down a gentle slope towards a beautiful beach, knowing that as you are getting closer to the beach, you are becoming more relaxed.

g) Once you feel confident doing visualisations, you can create your own inner sanctuary – a place where you feel safe and relaxed. The more you use visualisations, the easier and quicker it will become to achieve an inner state of calm and relaxation under *any* circumstances. This is your opportunity to play around with what works best for you, so you can enjoy your relaxation therapy.

h) Music is helpful and aids relaxation as long as it is in the background and it is calming music or some gentle sounds of nature. Listening to rock music is exhilarating and therefore unsuitable. Likewise, if it is music that invokes memories then that is not suitable, either. What you want here is to slow your thoughts right down so you can go within yourself to your inner sanctuary.

4. Once a state of calm and quiet is reached, stay in that place for a while. Remain quiet and go with the flow or introduce some positive affirmations. The following are my favourites for meditation:

- I am allowing my body to heal itself.
- I am safe.
- I am calm.
- I am relaxed.
- I feel energised.

5. If other thoughts come into your head, simply allow them to float back out again.

6. When you are ready, reverse your relaxation process by counting up from one to ten or by climbing the stairs

in your imagination. You should not use an alarm of any kind to bring yourself out of your meditation. If time is an issue, use a guided meditation or play a piece of music that lasts for seven minutes so that you will know when it is time to come out of your meditation slowly and gently. Alternatively, just finish when it feels right to do so.

7.   Finish by affirming that your mind knows exactly what it needs in order to do for you to recover fully from fibromyalgia/CFS.

8.   Allow yourself to enjoy the calm feeling for a couple of moments before moving on with your day.

What you can expect to experience

> Meditation is not a way of making your mind quiet. It is a way of entering into the quiet that is already there – buried under the 50,000 thoughts the average person thinks every day.
>
> Deepak Chopra

If you choose to listen to a guided meditation like mine, then you may experience various emotions that can come to the surface. Just acknowledge the emotions and allow them to drift away. This is a good thing, as it means you are releasing these feelings that you may have been harbouring inside for a long time. Initially, you will find that lots of thoughts come rushing into your head and that is fine – allow them to drift in and float back out again. Once you become aware of the thoughts, go back to your positive affirmations. It takes practise to quieten your often negative inner voice.

Meditation is a pleasant and natural state that so many of us never experience. Its benefits to your sleep patterns – and to your mental and physical well-being – can be immense. Do not allow yourself to be put off with false misconceptions that you will have to spend hours on end sitting cross-legged and humming. Give it a go for a few minutes a day – you might find you become hooked.

Summary

If you go to bed brooding over your day, worrying about the future, you are making it very difficult for your body to relax and drift into a deep, restful sleep. My strategy for a good night's sleep focuses on ensuring that you are in the best possible mindset for sleep. The sleep switch is designed to occupy the mind so that it is impossible to focus on negative thoughts. It will also provide a powerful anchor for sleep.

As you are climbing into bed, simply tell yourself that resting with your eyes closed is good for your body and think about all the things you have put on your gratitude list. This will calm your mind and remove any feelings of anxiety around sleep. Meditation will help you deal with every aspect of your condition and achieve the best possible mindset for living life to the full.

Key Steps to My Recovery

- Appreciate your day – relax.
- Trigger your sleep switch.
- Stop napping during the day
- Have a regular bedtime routine.
- Allow natural light to awaken you.
- Meditate to rest and rejuvenate in alignment with your circadian rhythms.

Chapter Seven – Understanding Pain

Life is like a game of cards.
The hand that is dealt you represents determinism;
The way you play it is free will.

Jawaharal Nehru

Introduction

Millions of people around the world live with the chronic pain of fibromyalgia/CFS lasting more than six months every day of their lives. This can destroy their ability to live a normal life and causes stress, anxiety, depression and decreased activity, which in turn often aggravates the problem.

The pain caused by fibromyalgia/CFS is very real and extremely debilitating; after all, who would want to move about if every time they did it hurt? My tender points were so painful that even the lightest touch was uncomfortable, so I struggled to rest comfortably. Add to this the muscle twitching and the sore skin, it is hardly surprising that sufferers become depressed.

There are many theories as to why fibromyalgia sufferers feel so much pain. It is my belief that it is caused by over-sensitisation of the nervous system, which amplifies and distorts pain. My protocol for dealing with the various aspects of the pain combine the very best of the techniques I tried. You will probably find that, like me, the improvement is gradual.

Terms Used to Describe Pain

There are different terms for different types and duration of pain:

1. Short-term pain is called acute pain.

Acute pain serves a very useful purpose in that it indicates the presence of disease or a threat to the body. Acute pain might be mild or intense, and it may last only a moment, or for weeks or months. In most cases, it disappears when the underlying cause of the pain has been treated or has healed and it does not last longer than six months. Many acute pains are like an alarm telling us something is wrong. For instance, if you were to put your hand on something very hot, you would experience pain. It can be caused by many events or circumstances, including:

- surgery
- cuts and burns
- broken bones
- labour and childbirth
- injections
- bumping into hard objects
- toothache and dental work.

2. Long-term pain is described as persistent or chronic pain.

Chronic pain continues or recurs over a prolonged period. It can be caused by various diseases or abnormal conditions. Again, the intensity may vary, but the length of time it continues often has a very negative effect on the lives of sufferers. Back trouble, arthritis and fibromyalgia come under this category.

Chronic pain does not usually present increased pulse and rapid respiration, as these reactions to pain cannot be sustained for prolonged periods. Chronic pain that cannot be treated medically becomes annoying and distressing for the sufferer. Persistent pain like this often serves no useful purpose. Sometimes pain can begin very small, but as the signals move along the network it becomes louder and stronger. It is a bit like tuning in to a radio station. In 1965, Mendell and Wall termed this phenomenon 'wind-up'.

3. Pain that comes and goes is called recurrent or intermittent pain.

This type of pain can vary greatly in intensity, as can the period of time it lasts. The nature of the pain can often make diagnosis difficult. A toothache would fall into this group.

Depending on the criteria, other terms are also used to categorise or describe pain. These can be confusing, so a simple explanation has been given below:

Nociceptive pain – pain is defined as nociceptive when the body's nervous system is working correctly, in which there is a source of pain; for example, a broken bone, a cut or a problem with the spine. It is the body's system of telling the brain that there is an injury.

Somatic pain – this is a type of nociceptive pain. The specialised nerves that detect somatic pain are located in the skin and deep tissues. They pick up sensations related to temperature, vibration and swelling in the skin, joints and muscles. This type of pain is experienced if you cut your skin, stretch a muscle too far or exercise for a long period of time. Nociceptors send impulses to the brain when they detect some kind of tissue damage. I can certify that this type of pain can be extremely intensive, as the surgery to remove part of my pancreas (to remove the tumour) meant that I had an extremely large wound known as a rooftop incision that was extremely painful at first.

Neuropathic pain – pain is defined as neuropathic when the body's nervous system is not working properly. While there is no obvious source of pain, the body nonetheless tells the brain that injury is present.

Pain travels from the peripheral nerves situated in your skin, muscles, bones, joints and internal organs to the spinal cord. These messages are transmitted in the form of electrical pulses. Once the signal has reached your spinal cord, chemicals called neurotransmitters are released, which then activate other nerve cells in the spinal cord to process the information and transmit it up to the brain.

Perception of Pain

There are many theories as to what causes the differences in pain tolerance, including ones that state it is genetic, psychological or even gender-based. But let's be honest – it doesn't matter how low or high your tolerance is, if you are experiencing discomfort it will be unique to you and can be extremely unpleasant.

The way in which we perceive something explains why two people can experience the same event, yet have a completely different view of it. For example, whilst I was in hospital I was given an insight into how differently we all feel pain. As part of my treatment throughout my entire time in hospital (approximately five weeks), it was necessary for me to have an intravenous drip inserted so that they could administer medication. This involved having a needle and then a small tube inserted into a vein. It was checked every few days and moved if the vein into which it was inserted was inflamed, uncomfortable or was beginning to collapse. I found it was only a mildly uncomfortable experience, but when a young woman was admitted to the next bed for two days of tests, she had one inserted and she actually screamed and cried. Then for the next two days she constantly described the pain as being level five – five being regarded as unbearable. Now you might be thinking this patient was a wimp or that there was another problem. But you would be wrong – it was simply that how we perceive pain and the levels we can tolerate are unique to us.

Perception, along with personal beliefs, is why you can have two people with identical illnesses or disabilities and yet their reaction to it and the way they live their lives and manage their condition is completely different.

Past experiences also contribute to how we perceive events. If you have been through a medical or dental procedure, for example, and it was incredibly painful, it is highly likely that the next time you have to have the same procedure you might be anxious or even scared. When a friend of mine had a routine inoculation that was extremely painful she became very frightened of needles for several years. In fact, it became a phobia in that she was even wary of sewing needles

100

and pins, refusing all future injections. It was only five years later when she was faced with no choice and was given an injection that she hardly felt that her perception of needles began to change.

Pain is a complex amalgamation involving our whole being and how our brain interprets the signals from the nerve endings. Part of this process is directly linked with the emotional centres of the brain. How we are feeling emotionally has an effect on our level of pain. That is why having a good laugh or exercising can strengthen our 'good' neurotransmitters and reduce our level of pain. Likewise, if we are depressed, angry, anxious or feeling down, or we are inactive, our pain becomes worse.

Endorphins – The Body's Natural Painkiller

The body has its own very effective painkillers called endorphins, sometimes referred to as 'happy hormones' because they produce a natural high. Endorphins are produced by the pituitary gland and the hypothalamus in vertebrates during various circumstances and they work as neurotransmitters.

The term 'endorphin rush' refers to feelings of exhilaration brought on by pain, danger or other forms of stress, supposedly owing to the influence of endorphins. When a nerve impulse reaches the spinal cord, endorphins that prevent nerve cells from releasing more pain signals are released.

Ways to get your own natural high

1. Sex

One of the reasons we feel good after sex is that after an orgasm we release a group of substances in the brain. Among them are beta-endorphins – the body's natural painkillers that give us that warm, relaxed afterglow.

2. Laughter

A new study suggests that laughing heartily with friends may help us to manage pain. An international research team, led by Oxford University, found that real laughter as opposed to a polite titter triggers the release of endorphins. It is important to note that studies have found that laughing when one is alone does not have the same effect. The fact that only this type of laughter releases endorphins suggests that it has probably evolved as a way of promoting socialising.

3. Socialising, chatting, gossiping

Socialising, chatting to friends and even gossiping (which I don't approve of) among human beings is the equivalent to the level of bonding achieved by apes and monkeys via social grooming. The Oxford-based Social Issues Research Council (SIRC) says that gossiping is a primitive need essential for our social, physical and psychological well-being. But I think it is the closeness and feeling connected to one another that make me feel good, not talking about others.

4. Exercise

Cardiovascular exercise including running, skipping, cycling and rowing, preferably four times a week for around thirty to forty minutes, is a fantastic way to release endorphins. Other nerve chemicals such as adrenaline, serotonin and dopamine are also secreted in the brain during exercise. These are required to produce a feeling of euphoria.

5. Spicy food

I cannot claim to have noticed this effect for myself, but it has been reported that this type of food, especially ones that contain capsaicin, like chillies, can trigger the brain to release endorphins because it thinks the mouth is on fire.

6. Chocolate

This is believed to stimulate your brain's pleasure pathways and cause the release of endorphins. Unfortunately, the effect of the sugar rush is short-lived, as is the effect of the endorphins, even leaving you feeling tired and worn out.

7. Music – such as classical and instrumental selections

It has been found that thirty minutes of listening to this kind of music releases endorphins that have an effect equal to that of the muscle-relaxer pill known as Valium.

Amazing Examples of Overcoming Pain

The body is truly amazing and capable of far more than most of us think. We have an inbuilt survival mechanism that allows humans to overcome astounding amounts of pain if their survival depends on it. Consider these next two examples of the survival instinct, allowing for individuals to overcome pain:

If you have seen the movie *127 Hours*, then you will know that in April 2003, after being trapped for five days at the bottom of a cold, dark chasm hundreds of metres below the Utah Desert, adventurer Aron Ralston amputated his own arm in order to save his life. After snapping the bones using his bodyweight and amputating his arm with a penknife, Ralston climbed approximately 20 metres to safety. He described the joy he experienced after he had sliced through the last tissue that had been attaching the useless limb to the rest of his body as being 'the most beautiful moment of my life. The intensity of emotion, the euphoria … It was ecstasy.'

Jonathan Metz, age 31, also tried amputating his own arm after it became caught whilst repairing his boiler. After being trapped in his basement for two days, he began to smell the stench of his own flesh rotting and believing it to be the only chance he had to save his life, he made the decision to amputate his own arm. Tying a tourniquet near his shoulder, he began cutting with some tools that he had to hand, but did not make it all the way through before firefighters, who eventually rescued him, finished the amputation.

There are many things that you can do to reduce your pain, some of which will also help other symptoms and are therefore covered in another chapter of the book. In this section we are going to focus on five steps:

- breathing exercises
- TAP

- positive visualisation

- thought distraction

- affirmations

Breathing Exercises

Fortunately, breathing is completely unconscious and we do not have to think about doing it. However, because it is completely unconscious, most of the time we are completely unaware of how we are breathing. Breathing exercises are a great way to release stress and tension. It is sometimes called conscious, intentional or transformational breathing. Essentially, they are the same thing: the conscious use of breathing to develop a very deep and relaxing state of inner consciousness. Meditators often use these techniques as a way to 'inner peace', health and vitality.

If you have suffered from mental, emotional or physical trauma you will have tension from stress stored up in your body. The effect of these negative emotions can be felt every time you move.

Benefits of breathing exercises

As we experience events in life there can be times when we feel threatened in some way. These threats can be real or imaginary, emotional, physical or mental – but they are all very real to us. Our natural breathing pattern can be changed by these fears.

In the past when I felt frightened, stressed or worried, my breathing became shallow, very rapid and high in my chest. Eventually, I experienced chest pains and would unconsciously hold my breath in an effort to calm down. Over twenty years ago I even went to the doctor because I was so concerned about the constant pain in my chest and was told it was the way I was holding myself. Apparently, I was tense and needed to learn to relax. I tried really hard but it only disappeared when I exercised or slept and then retuned very quickly.

Traumatic events that are not resolved at the time can remain in the form of contracted energy (cellular memory). This, in turn, can result in illness, depression, aches and pains in the body or in our case, fibromyalgia/CFS. Breathing consciously is believed to release this negative energy as fuel for the body.

Breath control is a powerful tool for connecting the body and mind. It has been used in various ways by disciplines as diverse as kung fu, t'ai chi, yoga, Christian monasticism and Kabbalah, to name a few. When we practise conscious control of the breath, we harness the power of the mind to the reactions of the body and create calmness, in turn reducing pain.

For centuries past, women have used controlled breathing as a way of helping to regulate labour pains. During labour the pain is often very intense. Breathing consciously allows the woman's mind to take over instead of her body. Therefore, she breathes slowly and deeply rather than the instinctive, fast, shallow breathing triggered by her nervous system. In other words, her attention diverts to her breathing rather than the pain. Thankfully, this technique works for more than just birthing pain.

How to breathe consciously

There are lots of books available on the subject if you want to study further, but this very simple exercise is the one I practise:

1. Begin by paying attention to your next few breaths.
2. Notice the speed of your breathing.
3. Become aware of where exactly in your chest you are breathing from.
4. Continue to be aware for the next few minutes.
5. Now pay attention to the quality of each inhalation.
6. Notice the feelings and sensations of breath flowing into your body.
7. Feel the places in your torso that move with inhalation.
8. Now pay attention to the quality of each exhalation.
9. Notice the sensations of the breath flowing from your body, the coolness or warmth of air entering or leaving the nostrils and how your shoulders drop slightly.

10. Begin to breathe in through your nose and out through your mouth, focusing on each breath.

11. Enjoy how relaxed you are beginning to feel.

12. Feel the places in your torso that move or do not move with each exhalation; for instance, the gentle rise and fall of your chest.

13. Close your eyes and continue to pay close attention to the ebb and flow of each breath.

14. As you continue to breathe, notice how wonderful each breath can be.

15. Continue to enjoy the feeling for a few more breaths.

I love the feeling I get from conscious breathing and the great thing is it can be done anytime, anywhere, and it is free. It is also a very effective way to calm both your mind and your body. It is particularly useful to bring the attention back to your breath in stressful situations.

Pain is never permanent.

Saint Teresa of Avila

TAP – Tap Away Pain

This exercise is based on TFT (Thought Field Therapy) and EFT (Emotional Freedom Techniques). It is likely to be different from any other form of treatment that you have ever used before in that it is unique. You may not understand how it works, but most of us don't understand how electricity works and yet it does not stop us from using and benefiting from it.

In brief, a key to the treatment is influencing the body's bioenergy field by tapping with your fingers on specific points of the body that are located along energy meridians. Acupuncture is an ancient healing system (at least 5,000 years old) based on the premise that by stimulating the flow of energy along meridians or pathways throughout the body, the body's own healing network can be activated. This technique also accesses the same energy system by tapping some of the identical points on the body into which acupuncture needles are inserted. I found it most effective if in addition

I gently tapped the actual points of the pain. This process also incorporates tuning in to the thought associated with the pain.

We feel pain as a direct result of the messages that are sent to our brain from other parts of the body. I believe that fibromyalgia/CFS sufferers are so tuned in to their pain that it intensifies, becoming unbearable and distressing. Tapping away the pain is so effective because it interrupts the signal to the brain and with this in mind, I adapted the techniques I studied so that they were most effective in relieving my fibromyalgia/CFS pain.

TAP exercise

When you are experiencing I pain, practise performing the following exercise:

1. Rate your current pain level from zero to ten – zero being no pain and ten representing the most intense pain possible.

2. Close your eyes.

3. Think about either what you believe was the initial cause of your fibromyalgia/CFS (car crash, illness or other trauma) or the emotions connected to the pain you are feeling. It is possible for the technique to work without this step, so don't worry if you cannot identify the initial cause.

4. Tap five times beneath each eye along the bony area. Note: all tapping should be done with enough pressure so that you can feel it, but not enough to cause you any pain.

5. Tap the 'collarbone points'. To locate them, take two fingers of either hand and run them down the centre of the throat to the top of the centre collarbone notch. This is approximately even with the spot where you would knot a tie. From there, move straight down an additional 2 centimetres. Then move to the left and tap this point five times. Repeat process on the right-hand side of the collar bone.

6. Rub the 'karate chop' point (situated on the side of either hand, below your little finger) five times up and down – ten in total.

7. Next, tap the back of your hand – about 2 centimetres below the raised knuckles of the ring finger and little finger when making a fist – five times using two fingers of the opposite hand.

8. Again, think about what you believe was either the initial cause of your fibromyalgia/CFS (such as a car crash, illness or other trauma) or your emotions connected to the pain you are feeling.

9. Open your eyes.

10. Close your eyes.

11. Open your eyes and point them down and to the left.

12. Point your eyes down and to the right.

13. Whirl your eyes around in a clockwise direction.

14. Whirl your eyes around in an anticlockwise direction.

15. Say three affirmations whilst tapping the actual point of your pain, (thigh, etc.):

    ▪ I am pain free and well.

    ▪ I am fit and strong.

    ▪ I am healthy and happy.

16. Count aloud from one to five.

17. Repeat the affirmations.

18. Tap the spot on the back of your hand again five times.

19. Tap the collarbone points again five times.

20. Tap the bony part beneath both eyes five times, one at a time.

21. Now, holding your head up, stop and check your scale of pain – note what your score from one to ten might be.

Repeat the process until the pain is significantly reduced.

Positive Visualisation

Your imagination is very powerful and the phrase 'a picture is worth a thousand words' is certainly true in the case of visualisation. Have you ever wondered why professional athletes and highly successful people use this technique on a regular basis? Well, it is a form of self-hypnosis and is a tool that can be used easily by anyone. By providing pictures (creative imagery) and through self-suggestion, visualisation can change emotions, subsequently having a physical effect on the body.

Advertisers are great at using images to fuel our desire for whatever it is that they are selling. Most of us at some time or other will have bought something we did not really need or have gone to get a snack in the middle of a movie after watching an advert for tempting food. By creating positive images of our own we are creating our own adverts – only this time for things we really want and need.

Our belief system is based upon the accumulation of verbal and non-verbal suggestions that have been gathered throughout our life formed around all of our experiences and our interpretation of them. Human beings see pictures on the screen of their minds when they think of things. For example, stop doing whatever it is that you are right now, close your eyes and think of your front door or your car:

- What do you see?
- What colour is it?
- What other detail can you see?

The pictures that we create are not like looking at a movie screen and can vary greatly from person to person. What actually happens when you think of your front door or your car is that you access a memory from your mind. When I consciously visualise I prefer to do it with my eyes closed, which helps me to improve the quality of the image. Even so, they are not sharp images – but this does not make them any less powerful.

When you visualise an outcome you want over and over again, you build cells of 'recognition' in your memory bank. This serves to help people with fibromyalgia/CFS greatly, because it means that you can become consciously and acutely aware of everything that can help you achieve the visualised outcome that you desire: becoming healthy and pain-free.

As explained earlier, everything is made up of energy, including you. When you continuously focus on an image in your mind, every cell in your body is involved in creating that image and you vibrate and resonate with everything that is in harmony with that frequency, both on a physical and a non-physical level. It is this frequency that moves you and everything that is needed towards you, for the manifestation of the desired image.

The brain is a highly efficient system that is connected to every cell in your body by billions of connections. Visualisation targets the right-hand, creative side of the brain to allow you to achieve your goals. When you visualise, you are directing unseen energy needed to manifest whatever it is that you desire. Everything that is created is done so in someone's mind before it is created in reality.

In healing, repetitive use of positive visualisation allows access to the mind–body connection. This enables the mind and body to work together to foster the healing process on a physical level. When you have an emotion, it generates a feeling that turns into a physical sensation. For example, if you are watching a horror movie, you may feel frightened and then get a chill up your spine, the hairs on your arms might stand up and your hands may begin to sweat. In this case you were getting a negative suggestion through sight and sound (your sensory perception), which would have produced an emotion of fear that turned into physical reactions.

Visualisation uses positive images to produce positive reactions or emotions in your body. Positive thoughts are essential to producing positive results. Negative thoughts and emotions lower the immune system, while positive thoughts and emotions actually boost the immune system. Many thousands of successful people have used visualisations to achieve goals – so give it a go.

First visualisation

In this visualisation you are going to call healing energy into yourself:

1. Think about the gentle warmth of the sun on a lovely summer's day.

2. Become aware of your breathing.

3. Begin to slow your breathing, focusing on each inhalation and each exhalation.

4. Imagine the warmth of the sun as a healing white light that is entering your body through the top of your head.

5. Allow the warm, healing light to flow throughout your body, all the way down through every part of your body, and connect with the earth – repeat ten times.

6. Now imagine the warm, healing light beginning from inside your chest.

7. See and feel the light getting brighter and radiating out from within your chest.

8. Think of it as a wonderful healing light bringing peace, tranquillity and joy as it heals your body.

9. Think about the warmth and brightness of the healing light as it begins to radiate out, spreading throughout your body.

10. Allow yourself to feel the peace and relaxation as the warmth and comfort heals your body, releasing pain.

Repeat this visualisation several times a day – or as often as is needed.

Second visualisation

In this next visualisation you are going to calm your nerve endings:

1. Become aware of your breathing.

2. Focus on each inhalation and exhalation, and begin to slow your breathing.

3. Visualise the amazing network of neurons that travel throughout your body from your brain to all your organs and down your arms and legs, all the way to your fingers and toes.

4. Notice the colour of this network of life – perhaps, as I did, you imagine it is red and inflamed.

5. Now focus on this amazing network beginning in your mind and send out a calm, healing colour from your mind – mine was a gentle, calm blue.

6. Notice how it starts at the beginning of the network and gradually flows down all the channels throughout your body, like a gentle, healing stream.

7. Allow the cooling, desensitising healing colour to flow or travel all the way through your body and all the way down to your outer extremities.

Repeat this visualisation several times a day – or as often as is needed.

Thought Distraction

Your mind is always busy and we now know that whatever you focus on you actually get or become. So it stands to reason that if what you think about most is pain, you will actually increase your awareness of your pain and probably the intensity of your pain. There are many ways to distract yourself and if it brings you relief for even just a short while it is certainly worth it. Some of them are more effective than others and their effectiveness will depend on both your mood and how bad your symptoms are that particular day. I am not suggesting that just doing something else is all you have to do to recover, but it is important to remember that this is a holistic programme of relief and management of your symptoms.

Ways to distract yourself from pain

- a good book
- crosswords, puzzles, Sudoku and jigsaws
- exercise – walking
- hobbies – painting, drawing, sewing, playing an instrument or computer games, etc.
- relaxing bath
- chatting to a friend
- grooming or stroking a pet

- music
- relaxation techniques – meditation
- watching a good film.

I used all of these methods depending on how I was feeling that particular day. It was important for me to have a variety of things to do to distract myself because, put bluntly, initially on some days I was not capable of doing most of them. Regardless of which one I chose to do, I always did it with a positive mindset.

1. A good book

Because of my symptoms there were days when I was physically unable to hold a book. But if I could manage to read for an hour or so it was a great distraction.

2. Crosswords and puzzles

This is a great way to keep the brain active. As I explained earlier, one of my many symptoms was brain (fibro) fog, so it was very important for me to exercise my mind and puzzles fulfilled this criterion. I chose very simple ones and on some days I would only do them for a few minutes. The idea was not to stress myself out thinking about what I could not do but to give me a few minutes of brain stimulation. If I only managed five minutes I congratulated myself on achieving this amount of time.

3. Exercise

Exercise is covered in detail earlier. However, often when I was in pain, I would spend a few minutes doing gentle stretches and balancing exercises. Not only did this distract me whilst doing it, but it would generally actually reduce the pain afterwards as well. Going for a walk was great exercise, especially if I combined it with walking with a friend, as it greatly lifted my spirits.

4. Hobbies

In an effort to give myself a relaxing hobby whilst I was ill I taught myself to paint using watercolours. It does not matter how much talent one has. Anyone can learn to paint and it is a lovely, relaxing, inexpensive hobby. There were days when I was too tired or in too much pain even to hold the paintbrush, but on those days I chose one of my other options. I actually exhibited and sold some of my paintings in the local art shop.

5. Relaxing bath

If I felt too tired and in so much pain that I could not even contemplate doing anything else, I would have a nice relaxing bath. The emphasis here is on the word 'nice', because it is not distracting lying in the water feeling unhappy.

> ☺ I would have lots of bubbles and listen to some relaxing music. That way, I found I could unwind in the warm, soothing water focusing on optimistic, pleasant thoughts and visualisations.

6. Chatting to a friend

Chatting to a friend or a family member can be a great distraction as long as you are not talking about your worries or symptoms, or theirs. Whilst it is a good thing to focus on the needs of others for a while, if you are the kind of person who feels the need to solve everyone else's problems then it should be avoided. I am sure you do not want to become the kind of friend who only calls to complain about how bad things are, so prepare yourself before the call – perhaps even plan the things you are going to talk about.

Before I started to recover there were a significant number of days where even the thought of actually having a conversation with someone would have been completely overwhelming. In fact, if I was alone I dreaded the phone ringing because I was too tired to hold a conversation. But if I did answer it and it was someone who was cheery and made me laugh, and who did not expect witty or stimulating responses, I would invariably feel better after the first few minutes.

> ☺ Once my recovery was under way I started to call friends and family. I was really touched how thrilled they

were that I had rung them for a chat and I realised how I had badly neglected some of them – thankfully, they forgave me. Now, I can be on the phone for hours without any neck or arm pain or fibro (brain) fog.

7. Grooming or stroking a pet

Stroking a pet has been shown to lower blood pressure, slow the heart rate, slow breathing and release tension in the muscles. It may even release endorphins – the body's natural painkiller and stress-reducer. Most importantly, animals are very responsive to affection and attention. Giving love to a little friend can alleviate loneliness and meet one of the emotional needs of connection.

8. Music

Playing cheerful music and singing along to it will always improve your mood. I had several compilations of really happy songs that made me feel great. I found that by playing them and singing along I could distract myself from the pain and how I felt. The only rule or guideline here is to choose any piece of music that makes you feel happy.

9. Relaxation techniques

Meditation is a great technique for relaxation and distraction, and can be done for just a few minutes as often as you like.

10. Watching a good film

This was the distraction I kept for my worst days, when I was incapable of doing anything else other than lying on the sofa. My world shrank drastically – bed, sofa, bed – but I did not watch endless reruns or reality TV shows. Instead, I recorded great films, series dramas or comedies and saved them for my really bad days so that if all I could do was lie down, I would regard it as a treat and enjoy what I was watching.

☺ Fortunately for me, my techniques worked very quickly, so once I started my recovery programme bad days were very rare. I actually found it was a nice treat to be cosy on a cold, rainy winter's day. Once something becomes a choice, our whole perspective changes.

Positive Affirmations

Before we look at how to use affirmations to effect positive change in your health, we need to understand the power of words and their role in your life.

As soon as we begin to understand words and start to operate as part of a family and wider society, we absorb words, attitudes, ideas, thoughts, feelings and energies from all around us. Many of these will be negative, because we live in a fear-based society.

The things that we hear as we are growing up form part of our early conditioning and this stays with us throughout our lives. Whilst most of us hear positive things as well as negative, sadly it is the negative things we hear and experience that have a much greater impact. Almost all of my clients can vividly remember hurtful or negative things that were said to them in childhood. In fact, many of them were so completely convinced they were true that it actually affected their behaviour and happiness for many years, until I helped them to deal with it.

Now imagine a world in which positive affirmations and words form the basis of our conditioning in childhood; think how different things would be. Thankfully, as adults, we can easily learn positive ideas. We can use positive affirmations to wipe out the old negative ideas, replacing them with new, fresh ones of our own choosing.

You can create your own positive affirmations, although for them to be effective you need to follow these guidelines:

- use the first person singular 'I' when saying them
- only use the present tense
- keep them simple
- say them with conviction and repeat them often
- be specific.

For example, if you just say, 'I want to be healthier', that is not specific enough. If you say 'In the future I will not be in pain', it will always be in the future. Also, keep to one area at a time. In other words, you would not combine 'I am thin and rich' – you would have two separate affirmations. In order to make it easier for you, I have listed some really good ones for you to use:

My healing affirmations

- I know that my healing is already progressing
- Every cell in my body vibrates with energy and health
- My muscles are repairing and healing
- My nerve endings are calm and relaxed
- I am healthy, healed and whole
- I am pain-free
- I choose health
- I naturally make choices that are good for me
- I take loving care of my body and my body responds with health, an abundance of energy and a wonderful feeling of well-being.

I know that some of you will be thinking but this is not true – I am in pain or I am exhausted. And I understand that, but the problem is that your body and your mind have learnt to do pain and exhaustion too well and what you are doing is retraining your mind through affirmations.

How quickly the affirmations work for you will depend on how much conditioning you have to overcome. For instance, if you have been suffering from fibromyalgia/CFS for many years and have firmly accepted the belief that you will not recover, you might have to repeat your affirmation like a mantra for months, whereas others might notice a difference very quickly.

You must be open to the concept that you *can* change your beliefs and you must also be patient and gentle with yourself if you are to work successfully with affirmations. Affirmations don't have to be said out loud. You can affirm them in your mind and that actually works better for some people.

We all have an inner voice and that voice for most of us is often very negative. If you think about your inner voice, you may find that yours is like mine was. Before I began to train my inner voice, I constantly told myself all day long how tired I was and how much pain I was in. What I was actually doing was reinforcing my symptoms.

Summary

In the Western World painkillers are so readily available that it is natural to turn to medication when you are in pain. But I found that unlike any other pain, no matter how many painkillers I took, they still did not reduce the pain. In fact, it was as though the pain increased in line with the amount of medication I took, so there was never any relief. My belief is that this is because my body was desperately trying to tell me that I needed to take action to deal with the causes of my pain and not just mask the symptoms.

My processes of dealing with the pain of fibromyalgia/CFS were far more effective and had no side effects. I am not suggesting that you stop taking the medication prescribed by your doctor or hospital, but you may wish to use my techniques in conjunction with medication until your need for prescription drugs reduces.

> NOTE: I strongly suggest that you consult your doctor or hospital before making any changes in taking prescribed medication.

It may seem hard to believe right now, but I know that through my processes I was able to rid myself from the terrible, debilitating pain of fibromyalgia/CFS and I am sure these techniques will work for you, too.

Key Steps to My Recovery

- Try the distraction techniques.
- Exercise sensibly.
- Use meditation to relax.

- Repeat positive affirmations regularly.

- Practise breathing exercises.

- Use the TAP exercise.

- Practise visualisations one and two several times a day.

Chapter Eight – Emotions

> Happiness resides not in possessions and not in gold; the feeling of happiness dwells in the soul.
>
> Democritus

Introduction

There is no doubt that the emotional aspects of fibromyalgia/CFS can be very distressing. You may even feel it has had a negative effect on your personality. It is totally understandable that someone who is in pain and feeling exhausted will be affected emotionally, perhaps feeling irritable and less patient with others. While most of us understand and accept this, some people with fibromyalgia/CFS get angry at the suggestion that conversely, their emotions, thoughts and behaviours also have an effect on their symptoms. Often they feel that it is insulting, almost as though it is being suggested that it is not a real illness, that they are in some way to blame or that it is a mental illness.

No one knows the real cause of fibromyalgia/CFS. But we do know that the way we feel, and our beliefs and attitudes, have an effect on our physical wellness and our ability to recover from any illness. My only concern was how to overcome fibromyalgia/CFS and live my life in a way that ensures I remain symptom-free.

☺ In fact, I was thrilled to learn that I was not reliant on the medical profession to find a cure in order to feel better.

It is important to manage your thoughts and feelings and deal with any negative emotions relating to your fibromyalgia/CFS. But it is more important to learn to manage your thoughts and feelings in everyday life.

When I was on the road to recovery I was concerned that if I faced a period of real stress my symptoms may return. It was only by learning to deal with my feelings and emotions, no matter how bad things got around me, that I was able to remain well when faced with having cancer. Since then I have been able to cope with many other challenges without relapsing.

You cannot always control the things that happen in your life, but you can control how you react to them. You are in charge of your brain and therefore your thoughts, reactions and results.

Your Emotional State

> The walls we build around us to keep sadness out
> also keeps out the joy.
>
> Jim Rohn

Have you ever wondered how one day you spilling your drink would fill you with negative emotions, like anger, frustration, etc., whereas another time it would have no emotional impact, you would just mop it up? If you were with a group of friends having fun, it may even make you laugh.

Most importantly, when you are feeling sad, lonely and generally fed up, your fibromyalgia/CFS symptoms will almost certainly be worse. On the other hand, if you are extremely stressed or frightened your symptoms may be temporarily disguised, only to return in the form of a fibromyalgia/CFS flare-up once you calm down or the perceived emergency is over.

Confidence, anger, fear, sadness and apathy are all emotional states which change throughout the day and how you experience these is unique to you. Put simply, your emotional state is your mood at any given moment.

This is very important because all human behaviour is the result of our state. Most of us are completely unaware that there is an internal process that takes place in the gap between the event and our reaction to it.

Everyone experiences negative states such as depression, anger, fear and frustration and if you are suffering from fibromyalgia/CFS, it is understandable that you will experience these emotions perhaps more than most.

Physiology

Although many people accept that their emotional state can affect their physiology or normal functions, very few people realise that the reverse is also true and that the way we use our bodies can affect our emotional state.

If you sit in a slumped position with your head hung for long enough, it will eventually affect your mood negatively and you will end up feeling depressed. Bad posture will increase aches and pains and your rib cage will start pressing down on the major organs, giving them less space to function. It therefore seems logical that if you use your body differently, you will experience your day completely differently.

Take a close look at your current posture. When you are feeling tense the natural reaction is to hunch your shoulders. Likewise, if you hunch your shoulders you will begin to feel tense. Most fibromyalgia (FMS) sufferers complain of terrible neck pain, which I believe is the result of hunching their shoulders. Consciously allow your shoulders drop throughout the day – even if it is only a small amount, it will make a difference to your neck stiffness and your mood.

Six Simple Steps to Save Your Day

When you are in pain and feeling tired, the automatic response is almost to curl up into the foetal position, hold your head down and withdraw from the world. The next time you feel like doing this you need to:

1. Stretch, take several deep breaths and fill yourself with energy.
2. Sit up straight and notice the good things around you.
3. Shake it out and re-energise yourself.
4. Stand and walk around for a couple of minutes.
5. Sing or hum a happy song that makes you feel glad to be alive.

Anger

Anger can manifest in many forms such as impatience, irritation, frustration, criticism, resentment, jealousy or bitterness. These are all thoughts that poison the body. When we release this burden, all the organs in the body begin to function properly. Anger can be a crippling emotion and it is one that a great many of us handle badly. When it is unresolved anger, perhaps with a spouse, a family member or a work colleague, it can aggravate fibromyalgia/CFS symptoms. Sometimes days, weeks, months, even years after an event people instantly feel angry or irritated if they think of an issue they have not resolved. Once they feel it is too late to go back and address the situation, the anger is coupled with resentment.

Women in particular often try to suppress their anger rather than express it in a calm and appropriate manner. At the other extreme, anger may manifest as shouting, which does nothing to resolve the underlying emotion and often escalates the level of anger. If you know you are too angry to deal with a situation, it is much healthier to walk away until you are able to still the emotion and then deal with the issue calmly.

During relationship coaching sessions husbands frequently told me how infuriating it was when their wives flipped over something really small. While the wives told me how hurtful it was that their husbands completely ignored their requests, until they eventually exploded! Teaching women how to express their needs in a way that men can understand easily often transformed their communication. Thinking about the outcome we want, waiting until we are feeling calm and expressing our requirements without laying blame is a great starting point.

Many people with fibromyalgia/CFS get angry with family members at the apparent lack of concern for their condition. Try to remember that watching those you love suffer and knowing you cannot help is a terrible situation to be in and often it is easier for the other person to try to ignore the situation rather than deal with it.

Tapping away anger

I read books about the power of tapping acupressure points and experimented with the exercises in them. However, while they had some effect, they did not calm me down quickly enough.

☺ People tell me it is my Gaelic and Celtic ancestry.

Thankfully, I was able to adjust the techniques into one that worked for me:

- close your eyes
- rub the 'karate chop' point on the side of either hand, below your little finger, five times up and down
- tap your chin five times
- tap your collarbone level with where you would fasten a tie on both sides, one at a time
- tap the back of your hand between the little finger and the index finger just above the knuckles five times using two fingers
- open your eyes
- close your eyes
- open your eyes and point them down and to the left
- direct your eyes down and to the right
- rotate your eyes around in a circle in one direction
- rotate your eyes around in the opposite direction
- recite a few lines of a nursery rhyme like *Jack and Jill*

(☺ I don't actually believe the choice of rhyme mattered; I just went with whatever came into my head.)

- and then repeat the exercise until you feel calmer.

Guilt

Many people have difficulty letting go of guilt. In fact, most people I speak to feel guilty about some aspect of their lives. They may feel bad about past behaviours or not being a good enough parent, spouse, child or sibling. If they are suffering from fibromyalgia/CFS, they frequently feel guilty about all the things they are not able to do.

I had things from my past that I felt guilty about, but thankfully I realised my guilt was just self-pity in disguise. If I was feeling guilty it was all about me and how bad I felt about my mistakes! So I decided to take action and deal with it. I believe this powerful step aided my recovery. I made a list of all the things I felt guilty about, decided where appropriate to apologise or make amends and took action. Then I thought through each situation and accepted that I had done my best at the time with the resources available to me. By resources I mean who I was at the time. The next stage was to forgive myself, with the firm commitment that I would be a much better person in future and that I would learn from my mistakes.

Make a list of your own past regrets over which you still carry heavy emotional baggage. Guilt can be a disabling emotion, often related to events from decades earlier that cannot be changed, so go easy on yourself.

☺ Yes, I did apologise to my daughter and husband for all the times I had been ratty. There were too many to address separately, so I went for one big sorry.

Fear

Fear often shows up as tension, anxiety, nervousness, worry, doubt or unworthiness. Some people believe that fibromyalgia (FMS) is fear displaying itself as extreme tension owing to stress and that in order to heal you must learn to substitute faith for fear. I am not just talking about religion – I believe in having faith in life, yourself, God, the universe and the law of attraction. You can choose to have faith in whatever belief best suits your model of the world.

In the past I lived a vast proportion of my life in fear. In fact, I was always afraid of something: being thrown back into poverty, not being loved, failure, ridicule, not being a good enough person, being hurt, the people I loved being hurt, losing loved ones, etc. My fears reached a critical point after my daughter was born. My love for her was so immense that I found myself spending much of the time feeling terrified something would happen to hurt her in some way.

Thankfully, I was able to overcome these fears completely and I realised that I was a resourceful person who could handle whatever came my way. By teaching my daughter to live her life with a feeling of optimism and happiness, she would be able to attract good things into her life and she, too, would thereby have the capacity to deal with any challenges that life sent her way. I could then relax and live life free of fear or worry.

Louise Hay (author of *Heal Your Body*, published 1976 by Hay House) states that fibromyalgia is caused by fear. Constantly living in fear will have meant that my brain and body were always on the alert for an attack that may or may not have arrived. This meant that I was continuously putting my body under unnecessary stress.

Fear directs, controls and affects so many aspects of our lives that it can prevent us from moving forward, in addition to having a detrimental effect on our health. When we perceive that we are under significant threat, our bodies prepare for either a fight to the death or a desperate flight from certain defeat by a superior adversary. This can be a very useful tool. However, all too often the threat we perceive is not real, it is imaginary. Fight or flight effects include:

1. An increase in heart rate, pumping up to five times as much blood to the arteries.

2. Constriction of blood vessels to the kidneys and digestive system, effectively shutting down systems that are not essential.

3.   Metabolism of fat from fatty cells and glucose from the liver to create instant energy.

4.   The release of endorphins, which are the body's natural painkillers. It is actually true that the hero or heroine in an action movie can carry on fighting even when injured because of endorphins.

It is no wonder that if you are constantly fearful, stressed or anxious – which can lead to full-blown fear if allowed to escalate – it will eventually have an effect on your health. To combat fear, the best strategy is to train yourself to bring your attention back to the present. Mark Twain once said: 'I have been through some terrible things in my life, some of which actually happened.'

My being on constant alert for problems was effective in its own way in that whenever a problem occurred, I would spring into action and deal with it to remove the threat to myself or my loved ones. Now, I am far more relaxed and I have faith in my ability to deal with things if they arise. As a result, challenges occur far less frequently.

> ☺ My husband has a great way of describing the way I used to be. He says: 'You were like a fluffy bunny rabbit with a machine gun.' I am still capable of getting angry, but it happens far less often and is generally appropriate.

Anxiety

Anxiety and fear both produce similar responses to perceived or real danger. Anxiety is perhaps recognised as fear but at a slightly lower level of intensity, producing butterflies in the stomach or a vague sense of unease. They are interrelated, as anxiety causes fear and vice versa. The following exercise is what I used if I was feeling anxious – in effect stopping the anxiety before it became a full-blown fear:

Anxiety buster

1.   Notice where the feeling is spinning in your body; it was usually in my chest. Emotions are energy, so the

feeling of anxiety will be moving. By focusing carefully you will notice it is spinning.

2.   Notice what colour it is – mine was usually dark grey to yellow; we are all different and whatever colour your unconscious mind chooses is fine.

3.   Notice which direction your anxiety is spinning in your body.

4.   Visualise it still spinning but moving up your body and out through the top of your head, so that it is now outside of your body.

5.   Change the colour. Some people see their anxiety as red and prefer to change it to a calming blue, but I instinctively chose a sunny yellow, so I went with that.

6.   Visualise it spinning in the opposite direction.

7.   Picture it going back inside you, through the top of your head, still spinning.

8.   Allow the calming colour you have chosen to spread throughout your body, filling you with calmness.

This exercise will help you to feel calmer by bringing your attention inward. Repeat the exercise in order to reduce your anxiety further. By practising this technique you will intensify its effects.

Forgiveness

When I talk about forgiveness people are often resistant to the idea. This is not because they are unkind but because they believe that by forgiving they are somehow helping the person who has hurt them in the past. Even worse than that, they are making themselves vulnerable to future hurt.

☺ Negative emotions become trapped in your body and are harmful, so let them go – you will feel great.

But it is possible to forgive without laying yourself open to more pain. This means changing your relationship with that person or maybe even ending the relationship altogether. Strange as it might sound, you can forgive but then move on. Holding on to bad feelings is like holding on to an energy-sapping sponge.

I firmly believe that the ability to embrace forgiveness and focus one's energies on the future is key to a happy and contented life. Feeling resentful and bitter towards someone is like 'drinking poison and expecting the other person to die'! I don't know who first said that, but it really resonates with me.

As a coach, I often meet people who are negative about things and they blame others for what happened in the past, which is actually ruining their now, their present moment and their future.

I had a client who was still angry about her divorce twelve years later. She got herself really worked up, talking about how she had not deserved to be abandoned and how bad things had been at the time. What she failed to recognise was that she had wasted the years following her divorce because she was more interested in being right and feeling bitter than she was in enjoying her new life.

My way of dealing with negative situations was to forgive everyone:

1. I made a list of all the things I needed to forgive people for in the areas of my life where I had suffered harm or emotional pain.

2. I worked on the basis that if I remembered an event with negative emotion then it should be on the list.

3. I sat down in a relaxed position and meditated on each one, visualising the other person or people involved.

4. I imagined explaining to each of them *briefly* how I had felt at the time.

5. Then I asked my unconscious mind what I needed to learn from this situation that would help me in future.

6. Next, I chose to forgive them. It can be that simple. We can choose to forgive or we can choose to continue suffering from our negative emotions.

I worked my way through the list, completing the above steps for each memory. Then I thought about each one again, making sure I could now think about it without emotion. I was not a bitter person and I did not feel that I held any grudges from my past, but to forgive was such a liberating and joyful experience that I now recommend it to all my clients and friends. If I could only pick one technique from this book to take away with you then it would be this one.

Try the above steps for yourself. Next time you are remembering something negatively, simply following steps 3 to 6 to see how you can change the way you feel.

Stress

There is good stress and bad stress. Some short-term stress – for example, what you feel before an important job presentation, test, interview or sporting event – may give you the extra energy you need to perform at your best. However, when you worry constantly about your job, school or family events, it may actually drain your energy and your ability to perform well. If you are suffering from extreme or long-term stress, your body, emotional state and health will eventually suffer.

Understanding your stress level is important. If nothing in your life causes you any stress or excitement, you may become bored or may not be living up to your potential. On the contrary, if large portions of your life, cause you stress, you may experience health or emotional problems that will make your fibromyalgia/CFS worse. Recognising when you are stressed and managing it can greatly improve both your life and your health.

Research has shown that many people with fibromyalgia/CFS have had a significant traumatic event in their past. It is my belief that the stress caused by traumatic events impacts on our health in many ways, including by developing fibromyalgia/CFS.

Identify your triggers to stress

In order to deal with and reduce your stress levels, it is important to identify what your personal stress triggers are first. Your triggers will be as individual as you are and the following list is intended purely to get you started on the process of understanding what stresses you out.

These generally fall into the following categories:

1. Emotional or Internal

These stressors are very individual and include fears and anxiety such as worrying about your illness, a lack of control over your life and feeling trapped or helpless. Certain personality traits including perfectionism, pessimism and suspiciousness can also distort your way of thinking or your perception of others.

2. Decision-making

For many people the need to make a decision sends their stress levels spiralling, particularly when it involves an important decision which is perceived as having a large impact on their lives.

3. Change

Not all change is bad. However, for many people change can act as a stress trigger because change means uncertainty and uncertainty can lead to fear, particularly if it is related to any important area of their lives. This may include moving, securing a new job, having a baby, a change in living arrangements or even going on holiday.

4. Environmental

Noise, pollution, lack of space and excessive heat or cold fall into this category. Even clutter can cause stress. Every time you cannot find something, stress levels can shoot up as you waste valuable time looking.

5. Illness

Short-term illnesses that are life-threatening naturally trigger the stress response as people are faced with their own mortality. Long-term illnesses like chronic pain and fibromyalgia cause stress for many reasons, including reduced mobility and the prospect of living with the condition for a long time. Some conditions such as herpes flare-ups are caused by stress; others like fibromyalgia/CFS are certainly aggravated by stress.

6. Physical

When one's body is overtaxed, it can be a trigger for stress; for example, working long hours without sufficient rest, depriving oneself of healthy food or standing on one's feet all day. It may also include premenstrual syndrome, pregnancy, menopause or over-exercising.

7. Chemical

Chemical triggers include excessive use of any drugs a person takes, such as alcohol, nicotine, caffeine or tranquillisers.

8. Family

Difficult relationships, bereavement, changes in a relationship with a significant other, financial problems, coping with difficult children, experiencing 'empty-nest' syndrome or excessively worrying about loved ones are all stress triggers.

9. Phobia

Triggers caused by situations people are extremely afraid of – such as spiders, flying in aeroplanes or being confined in tight spaces – can affect stress levels.

10. Social

Social triggers occur through our interactions within our social community. Again, they are very individual because they are based on our personal beliefs. For example, some people love public speaking whereas for others it is completely terrifying. For some individuals the idea of going on a date or to a party can be a trigger for stress. But for people with fibromyalgia/CFS, social interaction can become a stress trigger as the worry of how they will cope overrides any anticipation of enjoyment.

11. Work

This is an ever-increasing stress trigger in today's society. There can be a number of reasons the workplace can cause stress, including one's own beliefs. But it may also include the pressures of performing to meet tight deadlines, difficult colleagues, the fear of losing one's job and the demands of balancing work and home life.

To identify your stress triggers, write down the categories that the main triggers in your life fall into. It is possible that you have more than one or even many of the triggers. In an ideal world you would remove all of the stress triggers from your life, but it is often not practical to do so. Go through your list and highlight the ones you can eliminate.

Taking practical steps to reduce the stress in your life may, however, only have a limited result. Reducing the strength of your triggers is usually a more viable option than attempting to eliminate them entirely. How you deal with each area of stress will be individual.

Lowering your tolerance to stress

While I was working in the corporate world I fell into the trap of thinking that unless I could handle loads of stress, I was somehow not good enough! This is because in our society, particularly in the workplace, we tend to admire people who can handle stress. Some managers even refer to employees who go home on time as 'not being able to hack it'. It is a ridiculous statement where even if we are doing a great job, we are regarded as inadequate if we want to go home to our families. Ironically, it can even be seen as more acceptable if we hang around the office for an extra couple of hours a day, even if we are not actually doing anything constructive.

The fact is, you have as much stress in your life as you allow. Stop being afraid of admitting that you cannot handle everything. The more you take on, the more you will be given. These days I am often heard telling people that I do not handle stress well and I do not regard this as something to be ashamed of.

☺ As you may have guessed, I increased the stress in my life by the unrealistic expectations I had of myself, by being a perfectionist and by trying to control everything in my life. I am still determined and focused, and I have high standards, but I have stopped trying to be superwoman. As a result I am also far more productive.

Controlling stress levels

Start by recognising and acknowledging your stress level before it gets out of hand. When you feel your mind obsessing on negative events, it is time to stop, back off and regain your composure. You can do this by distracting yourself until you feel calmer, at which point you can then assess the situation by asking what action you can take. This is far more beneficial than going over and over it in your mind, allowing yourself to feel trapped. When you realise you are taking on too much and the pressure is building, it is a signal that it is time to re-evaluate things and slow down. Check that you are not trying to cram things in that are not important and discard trivial tasks where you can.

Your Inner Voice

Each and every one of us has an inner voice – the problem is that for many of us it is our biggest critic. We all know how crushing it can be when at a critical moment someone says the wrong thing. And unfortunately our inner critic is always around. Even when it is not putting us down, it is still increasing our anxiety by being negative. Indeed, the way we talk to ourselves can have profound effect on both our emotional state and our achievements.

Consider the following:

- Trust me to mess things up; I'm stupid.
- Everything is ruined; my whole life is a mess.
- This will never work for me; maybe it will for others, but not me.
- I am going to be ill for the rest of my life.
- I am never going to be able to live a normal life.
- I will never recover from fibromyalgia/CFS.

Do these sentiments sound familiar? The problem with these is that this is how most of us talk to ourselves daily. Because it is the voice in our head, we assume we have to listen to it and take notice of what it is saying. Even though one of the tasks of our inner voice is to help keep us on track and ensure we are making the right decisions, the way it speaks to us should be both supportive and constructive, like a best friend. Positive and helpful things your inner voice could say:

- I have the skills and determination I need to succeed.

- I am a good person; I will make the right choices if I take my time and trust my instincts.

- The techniques in this book will definitely help me to overcome fibromyalgia/CFS.

Notice what kind of negative thoughts are running through your mind and what you say to yourself that makes you feel bad. The following two exercises demonstrate how I retrained my inner voice that you may find useful:

1. Whenever you notice that your inner voice is becoming negative:

   a) Simply shout 'shut up' – it is just as effective to do this silently inside your head.

   b) Sing a few lines of a favourite song.

   c) Think of something positive.

   d) Then carry on with your day.

   Repeat tis process every time you notice that you have started running your negative thought pattern.

2. Change your negative inner voice:

   a) Notice the tone and volume of your inner voice. Is it spiteful, harsh, loud and intimidating? Does it sound like anyone you know? Does it sound like you?

   b) Focus intently on the tone and begin to change it. Make it whatever will sound the silliest to you. This is your inner critic; you can choose to make it slow

136

and sexy or fast and squeaky like a cartoon character.

c) Whatever tone you choose, make it sound as silly as you can, so that you cannot take it seriously and so it holds no power over you.

By practising these techniques, whenever you notice that your inner voice is being negative you will quickly reduce the negative effect on your emotions.

Media

Every day we are bombarded with negative news and images. It is enough to bring the spirits of even the most positive crashing to the ground. While you are recovering you need to stop watching the news and reading newspapers and magazines that are filled with depressing stories and features. I am not asking you to live in a bubble but to protect yourself from all the negativity around you.

I deliberately avoided listening to the news when I was recovering and I reached an agreement with my husband that he would inform me briefly of any world events he thought I needed to know about like an earthquake. This was great, because he would tell me what was happening without all the hype and sensationalism. If there had been a big disaster, we would make a financial donation and I would get on with my recovery.

This was not being callous, but I knew that I was not able to go rushing off to the other side of the world to offer practical assistance and I realised that constantly hearing about their suffering would not have helped me in any way.

I have never bought newspapers and magazines, so it was actually not necessary for me to stop reading them, but I would have done so because they can have a negative effect on your state of mind and recovery. So if you read articles about celebrity lifestyles, have a tendency to make comparisons with your own life and feel jealous or enjoy hearing about their misfortunes or bad behaviour, consider giving them a miss during your recovery.

Controlling Emotions

There will always be times in your life when you will have challenges to face. Regardless of the size or complexity of the challenge or crisis, imagine how wonderful it will be to be able to:

- control your emotions and choose your emotional state
- feel calm in situations where in the past you would have been angry or nervous, and
- deal with situations with effortless ease that would normally leave you feeling exhausted.

The following two exercises will help you cope with any situation that arises. The more you work on them, the more effective they will be. By practising them in advance and mastering your emotions before challenges arise, you will be much better equipped to deal with them when they do:

1. Calming visualisation:

a) Stand in a relaxed and comfortable position with your head held high.

b) Imagine that a golden thread is running all the way up your spine, out of the top of your head and all the way up to the sky.

c) Allow yourself to relax, feeling safely supported by your golden thread – become aware of your feet rooting you firmly to the earth.

d) Now remember a time when you felt totally happy, relaxed and calm:

- see what you saw
- hear what you heard
- feel how good you felt.

If you cannot remember a time when you felt at ease, instead imagine how amazing it would feel to unwind. Think of someone who is always very calm and in control and imagine what it would feel like to be them and how relaxed they would be.

e) Next, make the image more appealing by making the colours brighter and richer so the image is full of colour.

f) If there are any pleasant sounds, make them louder; but only to a comfortable level.

g) Allow your feelings of happiness, calmness and confidence to intensify.

h) Notice where the feelings are strongest in your body and give them a colour. Perhaps it will be a cool, calming colour or maybe one that you associate with happiness. Whatever colour you choose is just perfect for you.

i) Increase the brightness and then allow the colour to radiate out until it has filled your entire body.

j) Repeat the exercise at least three more times, each time adding more detail to the visualisation.

k) Enjoy the feeling.

l) Practise regularly to programme yourself to become more relaxed.

2. Calming anchor:

a) Remember a time when you felt totally happy, calm and relaxed. If you cannot remember a time when you felt at ease, imagine how amazing it would feel to be really relaxed.

b) Create the image in your mind:

- see what you saw

- hear what you heard

- feel how good you felt.

c) Next, make the image more appealing by making the colours brighter and richer.

d)   If there are any pleasant sounds, make them louder, but only to a comfortable level.

e)   Allow your positive feelings of being happy, relaxed and confident to intensify.

f)   When you are enjoying feeling relaxed, happy and calm, squeeze the knuckle at the base of the thumb of either hand using the opposite thumb and index finger.

g)   Continue to squeeze for a moment or two while you enjoy the feelings.

h)   Repeat the exercise at least five more times, each time adding more details to the event.

i)   Enjoy the feelings.

j)   Now think about a situation where you would want to feel calmer and more relaxed.

k)   As you are thinking about it, begin to squeeze your knuckle at the base of the thumb again.

l)   Imagine yourself reacting in a way you would want to.

m) Picture things going really well:

- see what you would see

- hear what you would hear

- feel how good it feels as things go as you would like.

- Make the image really appealing; make the colours brighter and intensify the feeling of calmness.

n)   Practise every day until you can recall the feelings of calmness instantly.

The next time you face a challenging situation, you can trigger your calming anchor by squeezing your knuckle at the base of the thumb. Concentrate for a few moments and access your inner calmness.

How I Stopped Worrying

Even though I am an optimist, if I had a problem I used to think about it constantly until I came up with a solution. Even then, I would continue to obsess about it to ensure my decision was right, going over and over every detail until I was certain I had not overlooked anything. It was as if I had no control over my life, so I was desperate to control situations I perceived as being potentially dangerous for me or my loved ones.

A big part of what I was doing was the need to illuminate feelings of uncertainty. One of the basic emotional needs is certainty and for many people, it is the highest need (this is covered in greater detail in the final chapter of this book).

I used to predict bad things that could happen in the future with surprising accuracy. But what I did not realise was that by doing this, I was actually causing them to happen via the law of attraction. To stop myself from doing this and to change the inbuilt pattern, I began to examine my beliefs about worrying by asking myself:

- What can one actually be certain about in life?
- Was the main reason that I was predicting bad things because I was uncertain about the outcome?
- How was this helping me?
- What good things might happen in the future that I was failing to notice?

When I realised that I was not helping myself in any way, that in fact if anything I was exhausting myself even more than I was already, I was then able to change my behaviour. Every time I caught myself worrying I would shout 'stop' inside my head.

☺ It is not a great idea to start shouting out loud in the supermarket.

Then I began to congratulate myself for all the things I had handled well in the past. I also started to trust in myself and in a higher power to take care of the things outside my control. We all have different beliefs and that is fine, but sometimes we have to let go and accept that we cannot control everything.

My top tips to reduce worrying

If you have spent many years becoming an expert at worrying, you cannot expect to become an expert at handling living in a calm and relaxed manner overnight. But you can begin to make changes immediately. Then every day, as you embrace a new way of living and realise how amazing life can be when you are freed from the shackles of worry, it will increase your enthusiasm for every aspect of life. As with every new skill, you start with the basic steps. My 'worry buster' will get you off to a flying start.

The worry buster

This exercise is designed to help avoid having a negative response by halting your negative thought process.

You need to *stop*:

1. Labelling yourself negatively for perceived current or past mistakes – I'm an idiot, I'm stupid, etc.

2. Filtering out all the positives of a particular situation or event – noticing the one thing that went wrong, rather than all the things that went right.

3. Emotional reasoning – I am feeling frightened, anxious or worried, therefore something must be wrong; I am in real danger.

4. Jumping to conclusions without evidence – I just know it will go wrong.

5. Always expecting the worst to happen – my husband is thirty minutes late; therefore, something bad must have happened to him.

6. Generalising based on a single negative experience, expecting it to hold true forever. You assume:

   a) one failed relationship means you will never have a successful one

b)   everything is good or bad with no middle ground

c)   if you cannot walk a mile every day you are not improving.

7.   Reliving the past or worrying about the future. No matter how many times you relive a bad situation in your head, you cannot change history. You cannot go back and make better decisions or react differently. Often, all we are doing when we focus on the past is torturing ourselves. If you truly believe something is likely to occur in the future, take action to mitigate the chances of it occurring. But constantly worrying, without good reason, that something bad may happen will not help you at all. You need to live in the present moment, because you cannot change the past and you do not know what will happen in the future, so dwelling on it only saps your energy.

Summary

Taking charge of my emotions was one of the most liberating and empowering things I have ever done. It literally changed my life. I no longer think the worst is going to happen or spend hours worrying about how I will cope with it if and when it does. I also no longer assume people will think badly of me.

One of my mentors told me that for the average person, 30 per cent of the people they meet will not like them for some reason or other, which could range from jealousy to not liking the sound of their voice. If this is the case then that is fine, because I realise I am no one's opinion of me. But to be honest, I view everyone with an open mind and assume that I am going to like everyone and that they will like me in return. This works really well for me as it means I am open to all the good that people can bring into my life.

I know that people can change in an instant and I witness it every day when doing breakthrough sessions with my clients, when their beliefs and behaviours change in just a few hours. But please do not be hard on yourself if you cannot change overnight, for your behaviours have been developing since the day you were born.

However, the more you practise, the quicker and the more amazing the changes and the results will be.

Key Steps to My Recovery

1. Ensure your physiology matches the emotional state you want to be in.

2. Use TAP to reduce anger.

3. Recognise guilt as self-pity and send it packing.

4. Forgive everyone – including yourself.

5. Lower your tolerance to stress.

6. Live in the present moment.

7. Whenever possible, deal with your inner critic.

8. Use the calming visualisation to control emotions.

9. Set yourself a calming anchor.

10. Use the worry buster.

Chapter Nine – Self-Esteem

Everybody is a genius. But if you judge a fish by its ability to climb a tree, it will spend its whole life believing that it is stupid.

Albert Einstein

What is Self-esteem?

The word 'esteem' is derived from a Latin word that means 'to estimate'. So, self-esteem is how you estimate, or regard, yourself. If you have a good level of self-esteem, you will be able to answer yes to the following questions without any difficulty:

- Do I like myself?
- Am I someone deserving of love?
- Do I think I am a good human being?
- Do I deserve happiness?
- Do I have good features/qualities?

A big part of this is recognising how your beliefs and thoughts affect how you feel about yourself, in turn affecting every aspect of your life.

Power of Beliefs

Beliefs are powerful because we tend to see them as the absolute truth and forget that they are just one perspective. Rarely do we consciously decide what we are going to believe. Our beliefs are an interpretation of events from the past, which can be incorrect or distorted, because a belief is merely a feeling of certainty about what something means.

If, for example, you believe that you are not intelligent, it is highly likely that you have negative experiences from your past to support this belief. A belief starts as an idea, like a chair without legs, and references that support the belief, like chair legs, to make it a whole.

Beliefs are the starting point from which we make all decisions. In moments of fear or pain they provide certainty. We are always looking to avoid pain and if we believe that falling in love will lead to us getting hurt, we may create the conviction that we will be alone forever. Convictions are extremely strong beliefs that often evoke strong emotive reactions when challenged.

Make a list of your beliefs and question them. Consider the following belief: The only way I will recover from fibromyalgia/CFS and my aches and pains is if someone comes up with a miracle cure. A better belief would be to say: I have the ability to overcome my fibromyalgia/CFS completely. How would your life change if you chose a different belief?

Beliefs can be so strong that in the case of people with multiple personality disorders, their beliefs may even alter their appearance. For example, their eye colour can change, physical marks may disappear and even conditions such as diabetes may come and go.

Limiting beliefs

When you have great self-esteem you feel like you can handle whatever life throws at you. You feel that you are good enough and that you are deserving of happiness and all the good things you desire. It means that you can appreciate your characteristics, talent and abilities without feeling the need to play them down.

It is not about being arrogant or showing off – these are actually traits of people with low self-esteem, because they feel the need to justify themselves and impress people. We have all met them and they are often extremely pushy, telling endlessly of what they have achieved or by trying to demand respect.

> ☺ I was raised with the belief that if I thought I was good at anything it meant I was vain or big-headed. Thankfully, I am how confident in my abilities and I enjoy them.

We all have limiting beliefs and in many ways they can keep us safe. For instance, if we did not have the limiting belief that human beings cannot fly without a plane or a glider of some sort then we may all find ourselves jumping off rooftops flapping our arms madly. But it saddens me greatly when people hold themselves back by their beliefs – usually because of low self-esteem. Examples might be: I am not very bright; I will always be overweight; I am unlovable; rich and successful people are arrogant; people like me cannot become managers.

If you have the limiting belief that you will never be able to recover from fibromyalgia/CFS, you should address that immediately. You may have given yourself reasons like: I have had it too long; I am worse than most people; my fibromyalgia/CFS is different; I have other illnesses that will prevent me from recovering. Whatever you have come up with, accept that it is a limiting belief, use the limiting belief buster (coming up) and take control of your life.

> ☺ Trust me – it will be worth it.

Many limiting beliefs come from the things that others say to us that we choose to take on as the truth or from an experience we have had in the past that we have chosen to interpret in a certain way. This is important because once we realise where a belief has come from, it is much easier to understand that it is not a fact and that it is just a belief; although it is not necessary to know where a belief comes from in order to change it. Finish these statements:

- The limiting beliefs I have about myself are ...
- Three limiting beliefs that have held me back most are ...

- I developed this belief because ...
- The cost to my life of these beliefs has been ...

Okay, that might have been a bit of an eye-opener for you, so let's establish some ground rules:

- Recognise that beliefs are not true; you are no one's opinion of you, not even your own.
- Your beliefs can be changed.
- If you feel these beliefs were dumped on you by someone else, forgive them – because they were not as enlightened as you are becoming.

The limiting belief buster

The following powerful exercise is for freeing you from the limiting beliefs that have held you back in the past:

1. For each of the limiting beliefs you have identified, write down the opposite of the belief, or what you are now choosing to believe instead.

2. Look at the people around you – friends, family and even people you don't know personally – who have made a good impression on you because of the personality traits you have identified in them. List the personality traits they display that you would like to adopt.

3. Now imagine you have overheard a group of people talking about you. What things would you like them to be saying about you?

4. Then write down the following:

   a) I am ever changing and from today the person I am choosing to be is someone who is ...

   b) The personality traits that I am choosing to show to the world are ...

   c) My old negative beliefs are ridiculous and stupid because ...

d) What I like and appreciate about myself are ...

e) The things that this old negative belief could cost me in the future if I don't change are ...

5. It can be difficult if you are suddenly going to become a new person with people who know you well, so the following tips will help you:

   a) Enjoy displaying your new personality traits to all new people you meet or to strangers in the street.

   b) Commit to displaying one of your positive beliefs every day.

   c) Be patient – you will fall back into old habits at some point. Start each day determined to display your chosen characteristics.

6. At the end of each day, write down the things you have done that best display the new you that you are committed to becoming.

Self-esteem is Vital for Happiness

Your self-esteem may have been affected by your illness or perhaps it was low before fibromyalgia/CFS set in. But if your self-esteem is low, it is essential for your recovery and long-term happiness that you increase it.

We all know that people who achieve great things generally handle life better than the average person. Their secret weapon is that they have greater levels of self-esteem and self-belief than the average person. They are able to call on these reserves at difficult times and thus overcome their challenges.

True confidence and self-esteem

If your self-esteem has been low for a very long time, you might not even be aware what great self-esteem actually is! How would you be like as a person if you had confidence and self-esteem?

Think about it for a moment and imagine:

- how you would stand or sit
- what your voice would sound like
- what kind of thoughts you would have
- what you would say about yourself
- how you would feel inside.

If you found that task too difficult then think about someone you know and admire because they are confident and have genuine self-esteem. Ask yourself the same questions about them and then imagine a new you behaving and feeling as they do. The more you practise this, the quicker feeling confident will feel natural to you.

How can you improve your self-esteem?

Accept that low self-esteem affects a great many people regardless of their success or outer veneer. So this is not another reason to beat yourself up – you are not broken or weird.

☺ Recognise that you are unique and special – there is no one quite like you among the seven billion people on the planet, unless you have an identical twin.

Nature made you unique, so celebrate. Give yourself respect and acknowledge your right to be part of an eclectic mix of society. Look for your special talents and use them to make the world a better place.

☺ One thing you have in common with all other human beings is that we all make mistakes – and that's okay! The key to learning is getting things wrong before we get them right.

Sometimes we feel we are 'no good' because of our past mistakes or perceived failures, but we have many aspects to our personalities and our current behaviour is just one of these. We are not our behaviours and as long as we are still living, there is always an opportunity for growth and change, providing we genuinely want to, and are prepared to take action to do so.

Increasing your belief in yourself – step one

Make a list of:

1. All the significant or challenging things in your life that you have achieved, coped with and handled. These do not have to be things that other people might find significant. Neither do they have to be traumatic or life-changing events. Growth is about gradually learning to handle bigger events and achieving more.

2. All the qualities you displayed in order to achieve these things.

3. The five things that you have achieved in your life that you are most proud of.

   ☺ I know for some of you this will be difficult because you fail to give yourself credit for the things you have achieved. But please try – it will be worth it.

Increasing your belief in yourself – step two

1. Think about a big change in your life or an event that you would normally worry about.

2. Imagine it going well – make a short movie of the event and run it in your mind.

3. Make the colours brighter, the sounds louder, until it is as appealing as possible.

4. Now imagine one or two smaller things going wrong and you coping with and handling them. If possible, picture yourself laughing loudly about it.

Increasing your belief in yourself – step three

Handling your biggest fear – for me this was a difficult one, because mine meant thinking about the loss of someone I adore. Although it can be challenging, it is worth the effort as it can free you from a great deal of anxiety:

1. Acknowledge the one thing you feel you couldn't cope with.

2. Now imagine yourself handling that situation.

3. What steps would you take to get through it initially?

4. How would you change or rebuild your life?

    ☺ Recognise that whatever it is you fear you would handle it – we always do!

5. Repeat steps one, two and three as often as you need.

I only needed to do step three once. I had a terrible fear of something happening to someone who is extremely important in my world and who I have sworn to protect – I guess you can work out who that is ... After years of fear and worry, I now feel certain they will live a long, happy, healthy life.

As your self-esteem improves you can start to make big changes in your life that will greatly increase your level of life satisfaction and happiness. It is important that you focus on the things that you *can* change now. This might mean starting slowly with small steps, but gradually you will be ready to achieve things far greater than you ever imagined. Even if there is nothing other than recovering that you think you want to achieve right now, you will still reap the benefits of better self-esteem that come from simply feeling good about who you are.

Accentuate the positive

Often we make ourselves unhappy because we go over and over past mistakes we have made. But you can improve your self-esteem if you rethink the things you believe you have done wrong or badly in the past. If after looking for the things you did right in the situation you still believe you made a mistake, then forgive yourself and learn from the experience.

Things you like about yourself

If you are seriously lacking in self-esteem then this next exercise could take some effort, but persevere and you will reap the benefits:

1. Write down your characteristics that you like.

2. Write down what you like about your appearance.

3. Write a list of your talents and skills.

4. Next, commit to writing down one more new thing you like about yourself every day for the rest of your life.

The Ugly Duckling

It is a beautiful summer day on the farmyard. A mother duck sits proudly on ten eggs. One by one, the eggs break open. All except one. This one is the biggest egg of all.

The mother duck patiently waits for the egg to hatch until at last it breaks open and out jumps the last duckling, which looks big and strong, but grey and ugly.

The next day the mother duck takes all of her little ducklings to the river. But the others all laugh at the ugly duckling because he looks different, which makes him feel sad. One day, he can stand it no longer and although he will miss his mother, he runs away.

Eventually, after many weeks of travelling alone and hiding from strangers, he comes to a river, where he sees five beautiful large birds swimming. Their feathers are so white, their necks so long, their wings so pretty.

The little duckling looks at them, yearning to be with them. He wants to be beautiful like them, but knows he is not. Then one of the swans calls to him to join them. Nervously, he approaches the water and sees his reflection. He is overjoyed to see that he is now a beautiful white swan. Happily, he enters the water and swims over to join his new friends.

Feedback and Criticism

If you have low self-esteem, receiving feedback can be absolutely crushing, but it is something you cannot avoid. If criticism is justified, it can be helpful if you ask what you can learn from it. If it is unfair criticism you can counter it by calmly putting your own case across and then forget about it. But most importantly, you can choose not to take it on board – just because somebody has said it, doesn't mean it is true.

Receiving feedback

Often when we feel criticised we are so hurt that we start defending ourselves without really listening to what is being said:

1. Listen to feedback without interrupting.

2. If parts are unclear, ask for clarification.

3. If there are aspects to the feedback that are valid, acknowledge and agree those points.

4. If you realise you were wrong, apologise.

5. If any of the feedback is wrong or unfair, smile and say, 'I'm afraid I don't agree with you, but thank you for the feedback.'

Giving feedback

Many people with low self-esteem avoid promotion at work because they cannot face the prospect of being in a position of authority and having to give feedback to others, fearing it will cause conflict or the other person to dislike them. Also, people show they are not in control and lower their self-esteem, only giving feedback when it is negative or waiting until they are angry before saying things like: 'You're incompetent'; 'You've messed everything up'. Statements like this make people feel out of control. They sound angry and accusatory, and usually result in an angry retort.

Fortunately, it is possible to learn how to give feedback in a way that people never feel criticised and actually positively take on board what we are saying.

The feedback sandwich

1. Keep calm.

2. Don't wait until you are too fed up or angry: give your feedback at the appropriate time – not days after the event.

3. Take three deep breaths.

4. Say something positive.

5. Explain what could be done better next time, not what was done wrong.

6. End with a positive comment.

General points

All feedback should deal with the behaviour or task, not the person. It should always be specific. When you are recovering from fibromyalgia/CFS, it may be necessary to let other people do tasks that you would normally do so that you can put your focus and energy into your recovery.

☺ This will be a great opportunity for you to forget about perfection and use the feedback sandwich if certain tasks are not done to your standards.

Relationships

People with good self-esteem generally have positive relationships, because our self-esteem has a direct impact on the quality of our relationships. People who have a lack of self-esteem cannot love themselves fully and will turn to the world for approval, hoping to fill this emotional void. Often, they believe that if they can gain the respect of others then they will have self-respect.

By depending on others for validation, they can become vulnerable, often over-analysing every fleeting glance and passing comment. No amount of respect and adoration from others will ever fill the void, because it is like trying to fill a sieve with water.

Bad relationships can lead to low self-esteem. This does not just relate to intimate relationships between a man and a woman but to other relationships, too. Generally, what happens is that one person will push their will onto the other person, be overly critical or generally display a lack of respect. Over time, this can undermine the confidence and self-esteem of the other person.

As Dr Steven Covey explains in his excellent book *The 7 Habits of Highly Effective People* (London: Simon & Schuster Ltd, 2004), all relationships are like a bank account. You make deposits and improve your relationships, but when you make a withdrawal you weaken your relationships. Unlike a bank account, the deposits do not just sit there – to maintain a healthy relationship you have keep making new deposits.

Your most important relationship

How is your relationship with yourself? That is a great question and often the true answer is 'bad'. We are so busy with life that we forget to look after ourselves. Even worse, we actually abuse our bodies and minds. Lack of self-care can come in many forms, from alcohol, drug or nicotine abuse to overeating and lack of exercise. Putting ourselves down and generally not taking care of number one, not having quality time for ourselves, can have a negative effect.

Does even the thought of putting yourself first occasionally make you cringe? At one time I was skilled at putting others first and for some reason covering it up, to such an extent that they were oblivious to the sacrifices I made. But not any more. It is not that I have suddenly become a selfish person – I love helping others and still do on a regular basis. However, I no longer forget about me and I no longer pretend I am doing something for me when it is actually to benefit another..

If you have ever been on an aeroplane, you will have heard the safety announcements telling you that should oxygen be required, you should put your own mask on first before assisting others. As a parent that concept is almost impossible for me to get my head around. How could I not help my child first? It was only after much agonising that I accepted that if I ensured I could breathe properly first, I would be in a much better position to care for my daughter's safety.

Life is much the same way. If I am fit, healthy and happy, I find it much easier to help others should the need arise. And because I now take the approach of helping others to help themselves, I don't end up exhausted as a result and they become more resourceful. Similarly, by not allowing people to take advantage of me, I am no longer putting my efforts into people who see me as a resource at their disposal. Both my feelings and my time are more respected and my self-esteem has improved as a result.

Being the type of person you want to attract

I believe the best way to improve your relationships is to *be* the person you want the other person in the relationship to be. By this I mean that if you want the other person in your relationship to be truly loving and generous, then be that person yourself. Never expect something of others that you can't do yourself. For example, if you are untidy, accept that those around you are likely to behave in the same way.

I am frequently told that other people are selfish or unloving, but when I ask my clients to give to the other person, without thought of expecting something in return, even thanks, they look at me like I am entirely crazy. But the fact remains that if you are only doing something for someone else because you are expecting something in return, then you are really doing it for yourself.

Undoubtedly, there will be some relationships that are destructive or unhealthy. In these cases, it is important to take a good look at the relationship and establish a plan of action, ending the relationship if necessary.

Energy vampires

Energy vampires could be all around you, especially if you are one yourself! Take a good look at the people you are attracting into your life, because generally people like people who are like them.

We have all met an energy vampire at some point in our lives. You are feeling great and happy and you are looking forward to a nice lunch with a friend, but within ten minutes you are feeling exhausted and depressed having listened to how bad the world and everything in it is.

Spending all your time talking about fibromyalgia/CFS or other problems, whether it be yours or other people's, won't be helping the situation at all. I know there is a belief that a trouble shared is a trouble halved, but in most cases the reality is that the trouble becomes doubled!

A client of mine once told me that she needed to talk about her illness because the sympathy was comforting – at least she knew someone cared. If you feel like this, ask yourself what you would prefer: sympathy or recovery?

I realise that because your friends are used to you being ill, the first thing they will probably ask is how you are, which then leads on to discussing your problems. However, as a client of mine recently discovered, people generally took their lead from her reaction. If she was bubbly and cheerful, most of them would be cheerful, too.

☺ When you are recovering it is important that you feel happy and positive – so beware the vampires!

Have you trained people how to treat you?

From the moment we meet someone new we begin training them how to treat us. For example, are we somebody to be respected, admired, pitied or abused? Unfortunately, many of us keep accepting poor treatment or behaviour whilst becoming increasingly resentful. We expect the other person to know that even though we are allowing them to treat us in a certain way, we are actually not happy with it. The other mistake we make is that we judge other people by our interpretation of their actions.

For instance, if you are someone who is normally very punctual and would never keep a close friend waiting, when your friend turns up thirty minutes late for a lunch date, do you automatically assume that you must mean very little to them? It may surprise you to learn that this probably isn't the case at all – it is just that they are bad at timekeeping and if you were to turn up an hour late, they would be fine about it.

Don't take everything on board

People get angry when someone rings up and tells them about their problem, because they suddenly feel compelled to sort it out. Instead of listening and showing empathy, they immediately feel even more burdened. They could choose to curtail the call and realise that whilst person has their sympathy, they are grateful that they do not have the same problem. Instead, they begin to obsess about it and get angry that yet another person has dumped problems on their shoulders. Resentment builds up and they find themselves asking: Do they not realise that I am ill? Why does everyone expect me to sort everything out for them?

I know that I have certainly been guilty of this in the past. I have actually heard myself offering assistance when I know I am too tired even to cope with my own life. Then I became resentful when they accepted my help. How can they accept? Don't they realise how unwell I feel? Well the truth is no, they don't. No one knows how you are feeling except you. And if you offer to do something for someone else, they will assume you are fit enough to do it and that you want to do it.

Practise saying no, particularly if you have someone in your life who is very assertive. It is best to start with something easy or small and gradually build up to the bigger things. You may find it easier at first to explain that you are involved in an intense recovery programme that requires all of your energy.

Everyone likes to be liked, but if someone's opinion of you is conditional on you doing things you don't want to then perhaps now is the time to re-evaluate the relationship.

> ☺ Whilst pushing my daughter on a swing one day, I remember watching two small children playing catch. After about fifteen minutes the little girl said, 'I don't want to play any more.' To which the little boy (her brother, I presumed) replied, 'Well I do,' and he continued throwing the ball to the girl, who kept catching it whilst moaning about being tired. Eventually she shouted, 'Mum, Tom won't stop throwing the ball to me.' To which her mum replied, 'Well you don't have to catch it!'

My recovery required me to be totally focused on my goal. This meant that I had to put other things on hold for a while. I also had to learn to say no to people who wanted me to do things that would drain my focus and energy.

This actually affected my relationship with some people, who did not like the fact that I no longer said yes to every request to assist them in some way. When I was first diagnosed with cancer I realised that those who I had always tried to help, even if it meant sacrificing my own happiness, did not care whether I lived or died.

> ☺ Like all things in life there is an upside. Although it hurt at the time, in the long run their rejection has been for my own good, because I now focus my energies on the many people who gave me their love and support throughout my recovery from all my illnesses. It is these relationships that have grown and blossomed, and I now find that I have more time, because I am not constantly trying to please everyone.

How to say no

People with poor self-esteem are always getting talked into doing things they don't want to do. This is because they fear it will lead to them being disliked, or cause conflict they feel unable to handle. If you want to say no in a way people will accept, stay calm, breathe slowly and speak without rushing or raising your voice. Use the word 'I'. Say, 'I'm afraid I can't make it to tea on Sunday because I need to rest.' Or, 'I'm sorry I can't work late tonight; I have other commitments.'

Once you have said no, move on and don't keep apologising or worrying if you have upset them. People who care about you will not want you to do things just because you feel pressured.

Forget About Perfection

The need for perfection and the desire to be perfect will often make you feel negative about yourself. Whenever you are obsessed with being perfect you are fighting a losing battle. This is simply because nothing and no one is perfect.

If you set yourself a goal and continuously focus on the fact that you have not yet achieved it, or you focus on any setbacks or slight imperfections along the way, it will almost certainly distract you from achieving your goal. Instead, focus on and appreciate the good things you already have in your life and then use these good feelings to help you achieve your future goals.

One of the most difficult things for people to accept is that relationships don't have to be perfect to be good. If you focus on enjoying all of your relationships instead of trying to perfect them, you will be amazed how quickly they improve. The way to become more peaceful is to deal with your negative and insecure thinking quickly. Take control of your emotions and ask what you can learn from even negative situations.

Have you ever noticed how stressed you become when you are caught up in a cycle of negative thinking? Or how you become absorbed in the details of whatever it is that is making you anxious?

When people have a problem they look at every detail of it, trying to analyse it from every angle, dissecting it and putting themselves through hell by going over and over it. This might be by going over the past or by worrying about what might happen in the future. One thought leads to another and they begin rehearsing conversations in their head. Often, they will feel that they are in some way the victim in the situation and that will inevitably lead them to feel less powerful.

I find it easy to spot when someone is focused on the negatives of an event when I ask, 'How was the party, wedding, holiday?' and they reply, 'It was good, but ...' Ask yourself how many times you have spoilt your enjoyment of a one-time event by focusing on the aspects that were not quite right, instead of focusing all your attention on what was good or great about the event.

☺ Don't try to be perfect – just be a great example of a good human being.

I have never had a policy; I have just tried to do my very best each and every day.

Abraham Lincoln

Don't Try to Change the World

Because of the amazing technology available to us, these days tragedies that happen across the globe are relayed to us almost instantly. Graphic details of natural disasters, acts of terrorism and wars are streamed into our homes. This can evoke a feeling of despair and a desire to change the world.

Every day people with extraordinary levels of commitment achieve tremendous success, wealth and fame, which can lead to a strong desire to make our own mark on the world. Most of us are not in a position to change the world and I think it would be very chaotic if we were all taking world-changing actions.

The good news is that we can still help to make the world a better place, while avoiding feeling frustrated and inadequate. We can do this by ensuring everything we do is with love and happiness in our heart. As Mother Teresa once said: 'We cannot do great things on this earth. We can only do little things with great love.' If we really want to make a difference to our world, in my opinion the best way to do this is to focus on the small acts of kindness that we can do right now.

Intuition

Have you ever said to yourself after an event: 'I knew that would happen'? How often do you know something is the right thing to do but then talk yourself out of it?

Trusting your intuition means listening to your quiet, supportive inner voice that knows what you need to do. Often, the only inner voice you hear is your inner critic that puts you down. Your intuition is best described as a feeling rather than a thought. It is not generally a conclusion you come to as a result of thinking something through. It is instant and instinctive. To be in tune with your intuition you need to be quiet and relaxed; meditation is a great way to do this.

Many people don't listen to their instincts because they feel the answers come too easily and so are too simple to be right. Another reason is because it often means taking action outside their comfort zone. Instead, they agonise over decisions even after they have made them and can spend many hours fretting over it.

Summary

As you begin to recover it is important that you develop the belief in yourself that you don't only cope but flourish through changes. You might find this a challenge at first, but believe me – the rewards will be worth the cringing you might feel as you admit you are amazing!

Constant belittling yourself definitely has a detrimental effect on your ability to achieve the things you want from life. Recovering from fibromyalgia/CFS using my techniques will certainly increase your self-esteem, because you will have the satisfaction of knowing you did it with the power of your own mind.

Key Steps to My Recovery

1. Use the limiting belief buster and increase your self-esteem with my three-step process.

2. Accentuate your positives.

3. Practise giving and receiving feedback.

4. Learn to say no and don't catch the ball.

5. Stop trying to change the world.

6. Forget about perfection.

7. Become the type of person you want to attract into your life.

8. Avoid energy vampires.

Chapter Ten – Diet

> The future depends on what we do in the present.
>
> Mahatma Gandhi.

PLEASE NOTE:

The information provided in this section is mainstream data that is widely available and is what I used to ensure I had a healthy, balanced diet.

It is not intended to be a substitute for medical advice. If you have any concerns about your weight or diet, get in touch with your GP, medical practitioner or a dietician.

Always seek medical guidance before following any of the information in this section.

Introduction

You might not think that diet and exercise have anything to do with overcoming fibromyalgia/CFS. But given that your body and mind are like a machine, it makes sense that you need to take care of them both in order to ensure that they perform well in all areas. Food is the fuel your body needs and exercise is like giving it a regular service.

Managing fibromyalgia/CFS does not necessarily mean that you have to eat nothing but cabbage and spend all day on the treadmill. It simply means watching what you eat and getting some exercise. Combined with the techniques in this book to deal with emotional issues and by making a few simple lifestyle adjustments, you will gradually begin to function normally again.

A healthy diet is an important part of taking care of your body and most of you will know what you should be eating. I am not going to start lecturing you about your diet or asking you to give up milk, oranges or anything else for that matter. Instead, in case you do not know what to eat to ensure good health, I will give you some simple, practical information that you can use to improve your diet if you feel it is necessary.

In my early twenties I was deeply unhappy. I felt like my life was out of control and I was trapped in a nightmare, emotionally unable to deal with my situation. I became bulimic for five years but thankfully, I eventually sorted myself out and adopted healthy eating habits. So I really understand the temptation to comfort eat when you are feeling low. But eating only makes you feel better on an emotional level for a few minutes and sometimes not even that long.

In the Western world, food is plentiful and it can be tempting to overeat. Often, people tend to use food to meet emotional needs but, unfortunately, it never works. Our emotions are the body's way of telling us that something is wrong. It is like someone knocking on a door – if we don't answer it, the knocking will just get louder.

Instead of overeating, identify the negative emotion and deal with it. The information and exercises in this guide will help you deal with your emotional issues in a much more productive way, so that food can become a source of fuel for your body rather than an emotional crutch.

Eating a sensible, well-balanced diet is always a good idea and being within the correct weight band for your sex, height and age will certainly mean you are not putting your body under unnecessary strain. When I developed fibromyalgia/CFS I did not have to change my diet significantly to deal with my symptoms.

For many years I have:

- eaten a sensible and well-balanced diet
- eaten my five fruit and vegetables a day
- had low-fat diet
- eaten sufficient fibre
- rarely drunk any alcohol, perhaps just a glass of bubbly at a wedding or on Christmas Day
- never drunk tea or coffee
- rarely have caffeine or carbonated drinks
- drunk 1.5 to 2 litres of water per day.

This did not stop me from developing any of the medical conditions mentioned in this book, but several doctors commented that how well I have cared for my body will have helped my recovery.

A Healthy, Balanced Diet

We hear so much often conflicting information about what we should and should not be eating that in the end we find ourselves not knowing what to eat. One year something is considered bad for us, so we avoid it like the plague, only to be told a year later that it is now considered to be good. My approach was very simple and that was to eat a balanced diet. Balanced simply means eating from all the food groups in sensible proportions. Now I am not claiming I stick to this religiously every day.

☺ People who know me well know how much I love chocolate – my one weakness.

☺ Oh! and ice cream – my second weakness.

☺ Oh! and curry – my third weakness.

On a serious note, generally I use my common sense. My diet is based on the following daily servings:

- fats, oils, sweets – eaten sparingly
- milk, yogurt, cheese – three servings
- meat, poultry, fish, dry beans, nuts – two servings
- fruit – two servings
- vegetables – three servings
- fortified cereal, bread, pasta – six servings
- fluid – eight glasses/2 litres of water a day.

A healthy, balanced diet contains a variety of foods, including:

- plenty of fruit and vegetables
- plenty of starchy foods; for example, wholegrain bread, pasta and rice
- some protein-rich foods such as meat, fish, eggs and lentils, and
- some dairy products.

A sensible diet should also be low in fat (especially saturated fat), salt and sugar.

Starchy Foods

Starchy foods such as bread, cereals, rice, pasta and potatoes are an important part of a healthy diet. Wholegrain varieties of starchy foods are the best choice.

I aim to make this food group comprise about a third of my diet. They are a good source of energy and the main source of a range of nutrients in our diet. As well as starch, these foods contain fibre, calcium, iron and B vitamins. I always try to include at least one starchy product with each of my main meals. So I start the day with a wholegrain breakfast cereal, a sandwich for lunch and potatoes, pasta or rice with my evening meal.

Starchy foods are not as fattening as you might think. Gram for gram, they contain less than half the calories of fat. You just need to watch the fats you add to them when cooking and serving these foods, because this is what increases the calorie content.

Fibre

Most people still don't eat enough fibre. Which is a shame because foods rich in fibre are a very healthy choice. I try to include a variety of these foods in my diet, such as wholegrain bread, brown rice, pasta, oats, beans, peas and lots of fruit and vegetables. There are two types of fibre – insoluble and soluble:

Insoluble fibre

Wholegrain bread and breakfast cereals, brown rice, and fruit and vegetables all contain this type of fibre. It cannot be digested and so it passes through the gut, helping other food and waste products move through the gut more easily. I love the type of foods that fall into this group, so ensuring they are part of my diet is easy. I never have breakfast cereals with added sugar and neither do I add any myself.

Soluble fibre

Good sources of soluble fibre include oats and pulses such as beans and lentils. This fibre can be partially digested and may help to reduce the amount of cholesterol in the blood.

Fruit and Vegetables

Most people know we should be eating more fruit and vegetables, but most of us still don't eat enough – I am lucky because I love almost all types of fruit and vegetables. In fact, I don't enjoy a meal if it doesn't include lots of vegetables. Once we expand our choices we find there is a great variety available. I always eat at least five portions a day. Snacking on fruit and vegetables is far healthier than reaching for the biscuit tin. By having raw vegetables prepared for snacking and a supply of fruit on hand, it makes it makes it much easier to make sensible choices.

For example, I have:

- a banana with my cereal; bananas are also a natural source of serotonin (the feel-good chemical), so they can help lift your mood
- an orange as mid-morning snack
- a side salad at lunch
- an apple as an afternoon snack
- lots of different vegetables with my evening meal
- a slice of melon or a kiwi as an evening snack.

There may not always be a vast choice of fresh fruit and vegetables available in the house, so in these instances I choose from my store of frozen, tinned or dried varieties. Fruit and vegetables make up about a third of the food I eat each day. I also make sure I eat a variety, so I get the best mix of vitamins and minerals.

Serving Sizes

> Never order food in excess of your body weight.
>
> Erma Bombeck

One serving = 80 g of any of these:

- 1 apple, banana, pear, orange or other similar-sized fruit
- 2 plums or similar-sized fruit
- ½ a grapefruit or avocado
- 1 slice of large fruit, such as melon or pineapple
- 3 heaped tablespoons of vegetables
- 3 heaped tablespoons of beans and pulses
- 3 heaped tablespoons of fruit salad
- 1 heaped tablespoon of dried fruit
- 1 handful of grapes, cherries or berries

- a dessert bowl of salad
- a glass (150 ml) of fruit juice.

Fish and Shellfish

I like to eat at least two portions of fish a week and I also try to eat a wide variety to ensure I get the best balance of nutrients – but I don't eat shellfish; it doesn't appeal to me. Fish and shellfish are good sources of a variety of vitamins and minerals and oily fish is particularly rich in omega-3 fatty acids.

Omega-3 fatty acids help prevent heart disease. Oily fish such as mackerel, sardines, trout, herring and salmon contain the richest source. The main shellfish sources are mussels, oysters and crab. Some white fish and other shellfish also contain omega-3 fatty acids, but not as much as oily fish. Fresh tuna is an oily fish and it is high in omega-3 fatty acids. But when it is canned, these fatty acids are reduced to levels similar to that of white fish. Although canned tuna is a healthy choice for most people, it doesn't count as oily fish.

☺ One of my speciality dishes is mackerel curry.

Although most people should be eating more fish for their health, there are maximum levels recommended for oily fish and crab, as well as some types of white fish. Please check with your dietician or health provider for the recommended amounts; this is particularly important if you take supplements containing vitamin A.

Eggs

Eggs (also pulses, nuts and seeds) are a good source of protein. They are easy to prepare and they contain both vitamins and minerals. It is important to store, handle, prepare and cook them properly to avoid food poisoning, especially for pregnant women, the very young and the elderly.

Eggs contain cholesterol and high levels in our blood increase our risk of developing heart disease. However, it is my understanding that the cholesterol we get from eggs has less effect on the amount of cholesterol in our blood than the amount of saturated fat we eat. People who are concerned about their level of cholesterol and who have a balanced diet should consult their medical practitioner or dietician.

I am not currently aware of a recommended limit on how many eggs people should eat. I enjoy eggs and think they are a good choice as part of my healthy, balanced diet. However, that it is a good idea to eat as varied a diet as possible. This means we should be trying to eat a variety of foods each week to get the wide range of nutrients we need. People who are concerned about their level of cholesterol should consult their medical practitioner or dietician.

Pulses and Lentils

Pulses such as kidney or lima beans, and chickpeas, are an edible seed that grows in a pod. Pulses and lentils are a great source of protein for vegetarians, but they are also a very healthy choice for meat-eaters.

Seeds

Seeds contain protein, fibre, and vitamins and minerals. They also add extra texture and flavour to various dishes and can be used to coat breads. Seeds make a healthy snack and I occasionally add them to salads, casseroles and breakfast cereals.

Nuts

Nuts are high in fibre, rich in a wide range of vitamins and minerals, and a good source of protein, which is important for vegetarians. They can be an excellent alternative to snacks that are high in saturated fat and they are a good source of monounsaturated fat, which can help reduce the amount of cholesterol in our blood. This food group also contains other unsaturated fats called 'essential fatty acids', which the body needs to sustain health. However, as nuts are high in calories, it is advisable not to eat too many them; salted nuts are very high in salt.

☺ Personally, I love most types of nuts, so I consciously have to restrict how many I eat – is this another of my weaknesses?

Meat

Meat is a good source of protein, and vitamins and minerals, such as iron, selenium, zinc and B vitamins. It is also one of the main sources of vitamin B12.

Cutting down on fat

Some types of meat are high in fat, particularly saturated fat, which can raise cholesterol levels. High cholesterol increases the chances of developing heart disease. When you are purchasing meat, always consider the type of cut or meat product you choose carefully. I always avoid fatty meats. I also remove any visible fat and skin prior to cooking because fat, crackling and poultry skin are much higher in fat than the meat itself. Other ways to reduce fat when you are cooking meat include:

1.   Grill meat rather than fry.
2.   Try not to add extra fat or oil.
3.   Roast meat on a metal rack above a roasting tin, so that the fat can run off.
4.   Try using smaller quantities of meat in dishes and instead incorporate more vegetables, starchy foods and pulses.

I mainly eat poultry and not just for health reasons; it is my preferred meat.

Fats

Ensuring that we have some fat in our diet helps the body to absorb certain vitamins. Fat is also a good source of energy and it provides essential fatty acids that the body itself cannot make. There are two main types of fat found in food:

Saturated fat

Eating a diet that is high in saturated fat can raise the level of cholesterol in the blood over a period of time. This increases the chance of developing heart disease. Foods high in saturated fat include:

- fatty cuts of meat and processed meat products such as sausages and pies
- butter and lard
- cream, soured cream, crème fraîche and ice cream
- cheese; particularly hard cheese
- pastries
- cakes and biscuits
- some savoury snacks
- some sweet snacks and chocolate
- coconut oil, coconut cream and palm oil.

How much is too much saturated fat?

According to information currently available:

1. The average man should have no more than 30 g of saturated fat a day.
2. The average woman should have no more than 20 g of saturated fat a day.
3. Children should have less saturated fat than adults.

Unsaturated fat

Choosing unsaturated over saturated fat can help lower blood cholesterol and provide the essential fatty acids that the body needs. As part of my healthy diet, I try to eat foods that are rich in unsaturated fat instead of saturated fat, including:

- oily fish
- avocados
- nuts and seeds

- sunflower, rapeseed, olive and vegetable oils, and spreads.

Trans-fats

These are found naturally at low levels in some foods such as those from animals, including meat and dairy products. They can also be found in foods containing hydrogenated vegetable oil.

Like saturated fats, trans-fats raise overall and LDL (bad) cholesterol levels in the blood that increase the risk of coronary heart disease. They are often used to extend the shelf life of processed foods, typically biscuits, cakes, etc. Any item that contains 'hydrogenated oil' or 'partially hydrogenated oil' is likely to contain trans-fats. This is why it is currently recommended that trans-fats should make up no more than 2 per cent of the energy (calories) we get from our diet.

> A crust eaten in peace is better than a banquet partaken in anxiety.
>
> Aesop

Fluids

Fluids are very important in order for our bodies to work properly and to make sure we don't become dehydrated. But to make healthy choices it is important to know what to drink, what effect certain fluids have on our bodies, how much we need to drink, what fluids should be taken in moderation and when.

Water and soft drinks

Water is a healthy choice at any time. Remember to check the labels of soft drinks bottles because they often contain hidden added sugars. Water is the best choice for quenching thirst between meals and for rehydrating the body quickly. It is entirely calorie-free and contains no sugars that damage teeth. Instead of drinking plain water, vary it by having sparkling water, add a slice of lemon or lime, or add some squash or fruit juice to flavour it.

How much water do we need?

In climates such as the UK, it is currently recommended that we drink approximately 1.2 litres (six to eight glasses) of fluid a day to stop us from becoming dehydrated. In hotter climates and when exercising the body needs more than this. As I rarely drink anything else and because I choose to exercise a lot, I personally drink approximately 2 litres a day.

Losing water

Water makes up 70 per cent of an adult's total body weight and without regular top-ups, the body's survival time is limited to a matter of days. It is vital for the body's growth and maintenance. Water is lost from the body through urinating and sweating, and must be replenished through our diet.

Signs of dehydration

One of the first signs of dehydration is feeling thirsty. People often confuse this with hunger and eat more than they need instead of giving their body the fluid it needs. If you think you might not be consuming enough fluids, check if you are showing any of these common signs of dehydration:

- dark-coloured urine and not passing very much when going to the toilet
- headaches
- confusion
- irritability
- tiredness
- lack of concentration.

Fibro (brain) fog can be much worse if you are dehydrated. When going on a long journey of more than twenty minutes, I used to avoid drinking beforehand because of the urgent need to urinate and this always led to a worsening of my fog. I have since discovered that not drinking sufficient fluid makes urine more concentrated, which in turn increases the need to urinate.

Thankfully, I can now enjoy journeys of several hours without any concerns.

Caffeinated drinks

Drinks that contain caffeine, such as tea, coffee and cola, can act as mild diuretics, which means they cause the body to produce more urine. Some people are more susceptible to caffeine than others, but it also depends on how much you drink, how often and time of day. If one of your fibromyalgia/CFS symptoms is the need to pass urine frequently, you should consider cutting down on your caffeine intake. However, reducing your intake should be done gradually, as cutting it out too quickly can cause side effects such as headaches. It is important that caffeinated drinks aren't your only source of fluid.

When I first decided to give up caffeinated drinks I was very concerned that I would be even more exhausted, having added occasional caffeinated drinks to my diet in an effort to give me an energy boost. But because I reduced my intake gradually, and replaced it with healthy stimulants like exercise and meditation, I actually found that I had more energy.

Tea and coffee

Most people love a cup of tea or coffee and there is evidence to suggest that some chemicals in tea may be beneficial for the heart. But tea and coffee also contain compounds called polyphenols, which can bind with iron, making it harder for our bodies to absorb it. Cutting down on tea and coffee could help to improve iron levels in the body. Tea and coffee have never played a part in my fluid intake because I don't like them.

☺ Actually, I have never even tasted coffee – I don't like the smell!

Milk

Milk is a very important part of our diet at any age. It contains vitamins and nutrients such as calcium and protein. It is good for your skin as well as being essential for healthy teeth, bones and muscles, and it doesn't cause tooth decay. For a healthy choice, I always choose skimmed milk. It is not a good idea to have flavoured milks, milk-based energy or malt drinks, milkshakes, or condensed milk because these tend to contain added sugars, which is bad for teeth and can be bad for the waistline.

Fruit juice and smoothies

Fruit juice and smoothies contain lots of vitamins that are good for our health, especially vitamin C. A glass (150 ml) of fruit juice counts as one of the five fruit and vegetable portions we should be having each day. However, we need to be aware that when fruit is juiced or blended, the sugar is released. Once released these sugars can damage teeth, especially if fruit juice is drunk frequently or in large quantities.

Fizzy drinks and sports drinks

Fizzy drinks, squashes and 'juice drinks' frequently contain lots of sugar, which means they contain a lot of calories and very few nutrients. There are low-calorie varieties available which are the ones I choose, but as they contain so many chemicals, I prefer not to indulge too often.

> ☺ I always choose the sugar- and caffeine-free options. In my model of the world, this means I can have more chocolate.

Alcohol

Alcohol is high in calories and so can make people put on weight. It is also a diuretic, which means it makes the body lose more water than usual, so it is easier to become dehydrated. Heavy drinking can lead to a wide range of health problems including cancer, liver disease, stroke and high blood pressure. It can also affect mental health.

I rarely drink alcohol and haven't done so for many years. For me it was a fortuitous decision to make because now that I only have half a pancreas, at least I know it is in good shape and will not have been affected by years of excessive drinking.

Please check with your GP, dietician or health provider for the recommended daily amounts. If you have drunk too much, you should avoid alcohol for at least forty-eight hours to give your body a chance to recover.

Vitamins

There are a wide variety of vitamin supplements available in stores. However, I prefer to get mine through the food I eat. Vitamins are essential nutrients that the body needs in small amounts to work properly. There are two types of vitamins – fat-soluble and water-soluble:

Fat-soluble vitamins

This type of vitamin is found mainly in fatty foods such as animal fats (including butter and lard), vegetable oils, dairy products, liver and oily fish. Your body needs these vitamins daily in order to function. However, you don't need to eat foods containing them every day because if your body doesn't need these vitamins immediately, it stores them in your liver and fatty tissues for future use. This means the stores can build up and become replenished so they are there when you need them.

Water-soluble vitamins

These are not stored in the body, so you need to have them more frequently. If you have more than you need, your body gets rid of the extra vitamins when you urinate. Water-soluble vitamins are found in fruit, vegetables and grains.

Unlike fat-soluble vitamins, they can be destroyed by heat or by being exposed to the air. They can also be lost in the water used for cooking. This means that by cooking food, especially boiling, we lose lots of these vitamins from the food we eat. I choose to steam or grill my vegetables most of the time because this is the best way to retain as many water-soluble vitamins as possible.

> The human body heals itself and nutrition provides
> the resources to accomplish the task.
>
> Roger Williams

Minerals

Like vitamins, these are essential nutrients that the body needs in small amounts in order to work properly. We need them in the form they are found in food, for three main reasons:

- building strong bones and teeth
- controlling body fluids both inside and outside cells
- turning the food we eat into energy.

Minerals can be found in varying amounts in a variety of foods such as meat, cereals, bread, fish, milk, dairy products, vegetables, fruit and nuts.

Salt

Every day twenty-six million adults in the UK eat too much salt. You could even be eating too much without realising. About 75 per cent of the salt we consume is already in the processed foods we buy. So if you are one of the people who put salt on their food before you have even tried it, try eating at least three mouthfuls before you add any additional salt and gradually reduce the amount you use to re-educate your palette.

☺ I always avoid adding salt to my food; although, I do enjoy a sprinkle on my porridge.

Vegetarians and Vegans

The important thing to remember if you are a vegetarian or a vegan is that you need to eat a balanced diet to ensure you are getting all the nutrients your body needs. Ask your dietician to advise you on the best choices for a healthy diet if you are in this category.

Healthy Weight

It is not a good idea to be either under- or overweight. Eating too much can make you overweight, which can lead to ill health such as heart disease, high blood pressure and diabetes. Personally, being a sensible weight where I feel fit, healthy and good about myself is important not only for my self-esteem, but also because I recognise that if I were carrying an extra 10 kg of fat around with me, it would adversely affect my energy levels, put a strain on my joints and make everything harder work. Not eating as much food as your body needs can also affect your health.

Overeating

There are many reasons that people overeat, most of which are not related to hunger. This is not a book about dieting, so I will briefly address the main three:

1. Boredom

It is easy to turn to food when you are bored. However, the truth is that if you are bored, your mind is actually asking to be occupied. There are lots of suggestions in the chapter dealing with pain for distracting yourself, which will work equally well for dealing with overeating through boredom.

☺ De-cluttering your life will also distract you from eating through boredom and it will improve how you feel emotionally – so it is a double winner.

2. Emotional factors

It is common for people to comfort eat, which means simply reaching for food in an effort to suppress negative emotions such as anger, anxiety, loneliness or frustration. Negative emotions are a signal that something is wrong and no amount of food will address the problem. The techniques in this book will also help you deal with any negative emotions in an appropriate manner.

☺ So keep reading – there is lots of help coming up.

3. Habit

Many people overeat purely out of habit. Often, overeating begins at a very early age and it can be a difficult habit to break.

My top tips for breaking the habit of overeating at mealtimes are:

- Weigh or measure your portions until you are in the habit of serving smaller helpings.
- Use smaller plates.
- Always leave some food on your plate at the end of each meal; this will break the unconscious habit of always clearing your plate.
- Eat slowly and consciously, actually tasting your food.
- Do not eat while watching television or engaging in another activity.

Under-eating

The exact effects of under-eating depend on the extent of the lack of nutrition and the degree of weight loss. Research shows that under-eating for prolonged periods causes health problems, including:

1. Heart, Circulation and Temperature

The heart can become weaker because it is a muscle that can be eroded by extreme under-eating. Blood pressure may fall to dangerous levels and pulse rate slows. Sluggish circulation can lead to ulcers on the legs, in addition to feelings of extreme cold.

2. Sex Hormones and Infertility

In order to protect more important life processes, sex hormone production is interrupted. Sexual drive can be reduced and menstruation affected.

3. Digestion

The digestive tract in under-eaters may slow down and as a result, food moves slowly through it and feels uncomfortable.

4. Energy Levels

The body makes energy from the food we eat and the oxygen we breathe. If we are not eating enough food and do not have sufficient fat reserves, energy levels can be affected, which when you are suffering from fibromyalgia/CFS will certainly make your symptoms worse.

5. Bones

Under-eating and nutritional deficiencies may cause hormonal changes, which can have a disturbing effect on bone growth and density. In later life the result will be osteoporosis, stooping and a high risk of fracture.

6. Skin and Hair

The effects of under-eating are variable from one person to the next. However, skin can become dry and show signs of early ageing. Some people find that their hair thins.

7. Sleep and Rest

Under-eaters may find it hard to sleep and may wake early with a sense of restlessness. If as a fibromyalgia/CFS sufferer you know you are under-eating, it is important you get professional advice on improving your diet.

The Marrow Contest

Of three contestants entering a marrow contest, the first man was lazy, giving his marrows very little water. The second man's tactics were to give his marrows twice the recommended amount of water and increase it every week, in the expectation that his marrow would grow faster and faster each week. The woman decided that she would give her marrow exactly the amount of water it required.

The first man was disappointed that his marrow was so small six weeks before the competition, but he was still convinced that his strategy was right. The second man's marrow had reached a magnificent size and would have won the competition had it been that week. The woman knew that her marrow was growing healthily and was satisfied with the result of her efforts.

The day of the competition dawned and the first man, who had deprived his marrow, was dismayed that his marrow was so small. When the second man went to cut his marrow, whereas six weeks ago it looked like a winner, on this particular day it had burst open and was beginning to rot. Neither of the men took their marrows to the show. The woman, who had taken a more steady, nurturing approach, produced a magnificent marrow and won first prize!

Summary

This is not a diet book and the information I have shared with you is from my own personal experience. It is not conclusive and therefore I suggest that if you have any concerns over your weight, diet or eating habits, you seek advice from a qualified professional. Try different foods; learn to enjoy cooking healthy treats.

My approach to diet is to eat the foods that I enjoy and make me feel good. By adopting this method, I feel satisfied at mealtimes and my energy levels are high as a result of eating foods that fuel my body best. Developing my sensible-eating plan was quite easy. As I am not a qualified dietician, I simply followed government guidelines and adapted them to suit my tastes and needs.

Key Steps to My Recovery

1. Eat a well-balanced diet covering all food groups.
2. Reduce saturated and trans-fats wherever possible.
3. Eat at least five portions of a variety of fruit and vegetables every day.
4. Drink lots of water and keep well hydrated.

5. Stay within the recommended healthy-weight band for your height.

6. Overcome emotional eating.

7. Deal with boredom.

PLEASE REMEMBER:

The information provided in this section is mainstream and is widely available. It is not intended to be a substitute for medical advice. If you have concerns abut your weight, get in touch with your GP, medical practitioner or a dietician.

Chapter Eleven – Goal-setting for the Future You Desire

> People are always blaming their circumstances for what they are. I don't believe in circumstances. People who get on in this world are the people who get up and look for the circumstances they want, and, if they can't find them, make them.
>
> George Bernard Shaw (1856–1950)

Goal-setting

It never ceases to amaze me how few people bother to set goals in their lives. It is almost as if they leave their future in the hands of fate and spend their lives living like an abandoned boat bobbing around on the ocean, going where the tides take it. Some people even spend more time deciding what to buy from the supermarket than they do thinking about what they really want from life and then wonder why they are unhappy.

Don't misunderstand me: I know there are unexpected events that happen – both good and bad. But generally I feel it is important to have a plan. After all, how can we get to our destination if we don't know where we want to get to? It might be enjoyable to go on the occasional mystery tour for our holidays, but generally we all want to know where we are going to be spending our holidays.

Alice Meets the Cheshire Cat

The cat only grinned when it saw Alice. It looked good-natured, she thought, but still it had claws and a great many teeth. So she felt it ought to be treated with respect.

'Cheshire Puss,' she began rather timidly as she did not know at all if it would like the name; however, it only grinned a little wider. Good, it is pleased so far, thought Alice and she continued, 'Would you tell me, please, which way I ought to go from here?!'

'That depends a good deal on where you want to get,' said the cat.

'I don't much care where –' said Alice.

'Then it doesn't matter which way you go,' said the cat.

'– so long as I get somewhere,' Alice added as an explanation.

'Oh! you're sure to do that,' said the cat. 'If only you walk long enough.'

Alice in Wonderland, Lewis Carol, 1865

Visualising the Outcome You Want Trains Your Brain

It has been proven that our brains cannot tell the difference between something we actually experience and something we imagine vividly. Just like a sports person who visualises success, you will improve your chances of recovery by spending time visualising yourself recovered. Mentally going over possible situations that may arise and imagining your strategies can help you become more relaxed and confident of your recovery process.

There have been studies done on the effects of visualisation in sports by some top universities. These clearly show that utilising the mind–body connection, whether it is through visualisation, self-hypnosis or affirmations, can significantly improve an athlete's skills. It can also help them to become more focused and even overcome or prevent training burnout. The difference between a mediocre and a great performance comes down to being in the right state of mind at the crucial moment. The ability to focus and block everything out that is going on in the world outside is key to being in 'the zone'. This is why many successful athletes use visualisation as a regular part of their training regime.

The Zone

We have all heard people talking about athletes or musicians as being 'in the zone', but what does it mean? When you are in the zone, you are in a state of relaxation, from which things come about effortlessly and easily. When you are in the zone you have total, absolute concentration, focus and single-mindedness of purpose, to the point that you are oblivious to your immediate environment. In fact, nothing else matters at that exact moment because you have switched off from your environment.

In the zone, performance of whatever you are doing is effortless as you become very relaxed. This means that you perform without taxing yourself mentally, physically or psychologically. For example, if you are working towards solving a problem, you will find that the answers come to you surprisingly easily when you are in the zone. Being in the zone also means that you are in sync with yourself: all of your parts are working together like one perfect unit or a well-oiled machine.

Being Realistic

People who live in fear will tell you to be realistic about your goals. This is because their past experiences and disappointments have caused them to have limiting beliefs. Individuals who achieve great things are rarely realistic by the standards of most people.

Mahatma Gandhi believed he would gain autonomy for India by peaceful means – many believed he was not being realistic but his belief proved accurate.

How to Set Really Powerful Goals

There is a tried-and-tested formula for setting really powerful goals that simply involves ensuring that you cover the right criteria. When you have fibromyalgia/CFS, getting well and recovering is going to be at the top of your agenda. In fact, I am sure that for many sufferers the thought of having any other goals while you are ill may appear pointless.

But I believe that having other goals can actually help your recovery process, because it provides purpose and a distraction for your unconscious mind. Also, when you are working towards a goal, your brain releases dopamine (the motivation chemical), which increases your ability to focus and motivates you to take action. As you near your goal the levels of dopamine in your bloodstream increase, especially if the goal is one that will meet one of your emotional needs. When you achieve goals, no matter how small, your brain releases serotonin, the feel-good chemical, which calms and soothes you. Basically, these two chemicals are your drivers, with high levels of dopamine driving you forward and high levels of serotonin providing the feelings of satisfaction, safety and comfort.

☺ I know only too well the dangers of setting goals on the wrong things or being too goal-driven, having passed a three-year course in just two years. So what I want to share with you now is how I set my goals and later I am going to tell you how I achieve them with very little effort.

1. Be specific

When I tell my clients to make their goals specific, they rarely manage it the first time. For example, if you set yourself a goal of I want to recover from fibromyalgia/CFS, obviously that is a great goal. But it would be far more powerful if you give it detail:

It is September of the year 20XX and I am preparing to go on a 5-mile walk. I am now fully recovered from fibromyalgia/CFS and I am generally in good health. I am symptom-free, I have returned to work part time and I love my new job ...

I could carry on adding lots more detail, but I think you will have got the general idea. It is well worth investing some time in ensuring you have sufficient detail in your goals.

A few years ago I was talking to someone who was pregnant about the forthcoming birth and I asked her what she wanted to achieve – her goal for the birth. Her answer was that she wanted it to be pain-free and over in five minutes, with a healthy baby at the end of it. Quite a good goal, you might think. But as I pointed out to her, there were a few things missing: in her goal she could have been at a bus stop or on a train without her husband with no other help at hand, for instance.

2. Congruent goals

When we want something it is easy to become so overwhelmed by that desire that we forget about all the other things essential for our happiness – like my own desire to be a full-time mum. For example, setting a goal of recovering from fibromyalgia/CFS and then taking a year to travel around the world would be an amazing goal – provided you had taken into account how it might affect other members of your family or your spouse/partner.

Many years ago I had a colleague who was very focused on retiring at fifty and he had a clear goal around this, which everyone knew about. He did retire before fifty, but only because of a heart condition. A better goal would have been: I will retire at fifty, fit, healthy and financially secure, and have the time and money to spend enjoying my retirement with my wife.

3. Measurable goals

If your goal is to make a certain amount of money, lose a certain amount of weight, pay off your mortgage or secure a particular job, it is easy to gauge your success as it is very measurable. But often the things that matter most to people are far more intangible. Yet, they can still be measured – you just have to know what you measure achievement of the goal by.

A goal is a dream with a deadline.

Napoleon Hill

When setting a goal of recovering from fibromyalgia/CFS, you need to decide what your measures of recovery will be. For instance:

- What physical things you will be able to do?
- Will you be able to work?
- Will this be full time or part time?
- Are you happy to accept some improvement in your health and pain level as sufficient?

I have lost count of the number of times my clients have told me that they want a better relationship with someone. But when I ask them what that means to them, often they are unable to tell me. The problem with this is that if you don't know how you are measuring something, how will you know if you have achieved it?

A better goal would be this:

> By December of the year 20XX I have a much better relationship with my sister, where we both contact each other once a week and we go out shopping or for lunch once a month. We have really enjoyable times together and spend most of our time laughing. We have resolved our past differences and both agree that it was no one's fault – we love each other greatly.

4. Time-bound goals

My clients often try to set their goals in the future tense. But the problem with this is that the future is just that – always in the future. So it is essential that you date your goal and state it in the now. For example, if you are setting the goal in March of the year 20XX to recover in six months, your goal should state: It is September of the year 20XX. I am ...

When setting my goal for recovering from fibromyalgia/CFS, I set it six months in advance, because this appeared reasonable to achieve. The date you put on your goal around recovery should take into account the level of fitness you wish to achieve.

I had a client who was very ambitious. She loved working at the company where she was but was unable to progress her career. She assured me she had set a very clear goal, which was: One day I want to be a project manager. A great goal for her to have – but just when 'one day' was is anyone's guess.

After our discussion she reset her goal to: In December 20XX, I want to be a project manager for the company I am with now. Within six weeks they had offered to give her the training required for her to take up this role.

5. Achievable goals

Goals have to be achievable or realistic – well don't they? But who is to say whether or not your goals are achievable? People around you will judge your goals based on their own limiting beliefs. Clearly, there are some goals that seem impossible even to me. For example, if I were to set a goal that within the next twelve months I would grow another 15 centimetres taller, this would be unlikely to happen as I stopped growing thirty years ago.

☺ In fact, if I did suddenly start growing again, I might be a bit concerned.

But if I decided I was going to become a nuclear scientist, as long as I gave myself sufficient time and the motivation to do something about it, it would be achievable.

Then there is the other extreme, where people are too tied to their beliefs that life is meant to be difficult, that they are not meant to be happy or that they are unable to change. I have already covered limiting beliefs, so by now you should be aware of yours and how to deal with them. If not, I suggest you go back and look at the chapter on self-esteem.

All too often my clients tell me that they always wanted to achieve something – a fulfilling career or a great relationship, for instance – but they have never even tried because they honestly don't believe they could achieve it or, even worse, they believe that they don't deserve it.

I don't believe anyone should be held back by their own or by anyone else's beliefs in their abilities. I also don't think success always has to mean a struggle and hard work, but you definitely have to be prepared to take action. Unfortunately, if you announce that you are going to make a million pounds in the next year and then spend twelve hours a day watching television, this goal is unlikely to be achievable.

☺ Unless that is part of your strategy and perhaps you are writing screenplays.

Your goals have to be big enough to motivate you to take action and to keep you focused when other things might distract you from achieving them. Success-coaching guru Antony Robbins says: 'Make your goals so big that they make your problems appear insignificant by comparison'. So please go beyond what you currently think you can achieve – be optimistic.

What is really important, though, is that your goals are realistic to you and that you actually believe you have a chance of achieving them. If the goal you have thought of appears too big or too far away and out of reach, it will be difficult to stay motivated. You can overcome this by setting yourself smaller goals that you can achieve along the way to your bigger dream and by working on your limiting beliefs about yourself.

The Four-Minute Mile

For many years it was widely believed to be impossible for a human to run a mile (1,609 metres) in under four minutes. In fact, for many years it was believed that the four-minute mile was a physical barrier that no man or woman could break without causing significant damage to the runner's health, the belief being that their lungs might explode or their heart would give up. The achievement of a four-minute mile seemed beyond human possibility.

On 6 May 1954, during an athletic meeting, Roger Bannister ran a mile in 3 minutes and 59.4 seconds and broke the 'four-minute mile' psychological barrier. Then fifty-six days later John Landy ran the four-minute mile in 3 minutes and 57.9 seconds in Finland. In the coming months and years many others followed their example, breaking their own four-minute miles.

The Law of Attraction

Many authors have written books on the law of attraction and have done so far better than I could, so my explanation of it will be brief. However, this should not detract from the massive importance I place on my beliefs around the law of attraction and its power to attract both good and bad things into my life.

If you look at any of the religions of the world, you can find the law of attraction delivered through its stories. Many of the world's greatest teachers, artists and thinkers have shared its message through their teaching.

> ☺ I am going to start by sharing what I have read and understood about it. Then I will share my personal beliefs.

Your thoughts and emotions are magnetic and have a frequency. As you think, your thoughts are sent out into the universe, attracting to you things that are transmitting on the same frequency. In other words, thoughts become things.

Put simply, what you think about most you attract to you. At first this might be difficult for you to accept, but the law of attraction states that everything in your life right now has been attracted to you, by you.

> ☺ Please don't shout at me – I did not invent this concept. All I know is that in my case, certainly as an adult, it is true. I accept 100 per cent that everything in my life, including my illnesses, has happened as a result of conscious or unconscious decisions I have made or beliefs I have held.

What you think, you become. A person who constantly thinks angry or bitter thoughts becomes a bitter and angry person. If you are thinking angry thoughts, you are holding them in your heart and so you will attract more things to you to make you feel angry.

I watched a TV show recently that was based on a true story. It was about a prisoner of war who pretended to be insane over a period of eighteen months in order to be repatriated. Indeed, he managed to convince everyone of his insanity by keeping up his pretence on a constant basis. Eventually, he was repatriated and his fellow prisoners rejoiced, until they heard from his wife that he had been admitted to a mental institution. Unfortunately his act had been so good that he had convinced himself he *was* insane and therefore become that person.

Okay, now this next part is for the more practical amongst you. I have taught this to hundreds of clients who have been amazed at the results.

> ☺ Even my teenage daughter is impressed at what she achieves by using this methodology of thinking positively.

I like to think that the universe is connected by magnetic forces because I think it is such an amazing concept. But when I am feeling more grounded, I know that the unconscious mind is constantly working to deliver me the things I think about and want most. So it is very easy for me to accept that if I think about something, my unconscious mind assumes it is something I desire and therefore gives me instructions so that I find myself instinctively taking actions to deliver me what I want.

My belief in the law of attraction and my ability to use the strategy enable me to achieve all my goals with ease. This does not mean that I don't put in any effort or take action. What this means is that all my actions are instinctively targeted towards achieving my goals.

I would hate for anyone to think that their thoughts in some way contributed to the loss of a loved one or a loved one being hurt in some way. So please be assured that you are not responsible for what happens to others and you cannot cause bad things to happen in someone else's life.

We know from various studies that your mind processes everything as a positive first. For instance, if I say 'Don't think of a blue tree,' you automatically have to think about it. It is impossible not to, even if it is only for a second. You have to think about it before you reach a point where you decide that you cannot or shouldn't do so.

So how can you retrain your brain to think about the things you want? By this I do not mean sitting back and thinking: I want to get well and have a million pounds and expecting it to happen. You have to know what you want, tell your unconscious mind what you want and then be willing to take action guided by your unconscious mind so that you can achieve your goal. In simple terms, it means having a clear positive image, following your positive instincts, monitoring your results, and changing your thoughts and actions as needed.

The science of the law of attraction

From a psychological point of view, the law of attraction is best explained as the information-filtering system of the brain known as the reticular activating system (RAS). At the base of the human brainstem there is a small, finger-sized control centre called the RAS that evaluates incoming data.

A simple way to explain your RAS is that it is responsible for filtering incoming information that your brain receives and it also acts as a receiver for information that is tagged as being important. Think of it like a radio: you are surrounded by radio waves from a large number of stations but your radio can only pick up one of these channels at a time. In order to hear your chosen station clearly, you have to tune in to it. Your RAS is similar. If you are in a room talking to several people and engaged in a conversation on one side of the room, when on the other side of the room your name is mentioned, at this point all your attention will be diverted in the direction that you heard your name. This is because that bit of information is tagged by the RAS as being important to you.

The RAS is what enables a parent to sleep through various familiar noises but wake instantly if their baby makes the smallest cry. I remember Mum always said my eldest sister would sleep through a rock concert, but once my niece was born she instinctively woke at even the slightest sound. This is because the RAS is naturally programmed to prioritise information that is necessary for survival;

for instance, listening for the sound of an oncoming vehicle when crossing the road. However, the RAS does not distinguish between a real event and a contrived reality. This means we can use this to our advantage by programming it to seek out stimuli in our environment that resonate with our goals.

The process of creating a vision board is one of the best ways to programme the RAS, by stimulating it to pay attention to certain things in your environment that are in frequency with your goal or vision. It works in much the same way as you are able to pick up your name being mentioned in a conversation on the other side of a room, while at the same time talking to others. This selective attention filter makes you aware of daily things that can help you achieve your goal and it is your job to take action on those opportunities when they present themselves.

What is a vision board?

A vision board is a very powerful yet simple visualisation tool that helps activate the universal law of attraction into manifesting your dreams into reality. This concept has been around for generations and is also known as a goal board, goal map or treasure map.

It is simply a visual representation or collage of the things that you want to have, be or do in your life. The purpose of your vision board is to activate the law or attraction or stimulate your RAS (whichever you choose to believe and gets you the best results) to begin to attract things from your external environment that will enable you to realise your goals. By selecting powerful pictures and words that stimulate the positive emotions of passion and motivation, you will begin to manifest those things into your life.

Elements of a good vision board

1. Visual

The unconscious mind works in pictures and images, so make your vision board as visual as possible with as many pictures as you can. The images can be supplemented with inspiring words and phrases. Both the pictures and the words should very closely represent your desires. So when creating a vision board use images that clearly state your recovery from fibromyalgia/CFS, and you achieving great health and having the life you want. For example, if you like the idea of being able to go on a walking holiday to a particular country, choose images that will represent this to you.

☺ If you want a Labrador and put a picture of a Yorkshire terrier on your board, don't be surprised to find yourself with a little Yorkie very soon. But Yorkies are adorable!

2. Emotional

All the pictures on your vision board should evoke a positive emotional response from you. Just looking at your vision board should fuel your passion to achieve the images and make you feel happy every time you look at it.

Positioning your board

Criticism from others may lead to self-doubt and negativity, which will damage the delicate energy that your vision board emits. So if you are concerned that others will criticise or mock your board, place it in a private location so it can only be seen by you. Ideally, your board should be situated in a location where you will see it often, giving your unconscious mind maximum exposure to it, thereby enabling you to achieve your desires far quicker than you might currently imagine.

The Midas Touch

The King of Phrygia was known as Midas. He was a very kind man who ruled his kingdom fairly, but he was not one to think very deeply about what he said. He was a very wealthy man, and had riches that most people would have felt very fortunate to have, but Midas still desired more wealth.

One day while walking in the beautiful grounds of his house, when passing through a blaze of colour and intoxicating fragrance, he saw an elderly man asleep in the flowers. King Midas realised that the old man was unwell. Taking pity on the old fellow, he ordered the guards to help him to his feet and make him welcome in the palace until he recovered.

When the gods heard about it, they rewarded this kindness by granting Midas one wish. The king thought for only a second and then said, 'I wish for everything I touch to turn to gold.'

'If you are you sure that is what you want,' said the gods, knowing that it was a foolish wish that Midas might live to regret. And so it was.

Midas could hardly wait to put his new skill to the test and so he touched a chair, a table and then a book, all instantly turning to gold. He could hardly control his excitement and ran out into the garden, brushing all the flowers as he passed then, which immediately turned rigid and gold.

Overjoyed, King Midas ordered a great banquet in celebration. However, as soon as he touched the food it, too, turned to solid gold, his wine turning to liquid gold, and the king realised to his horror what he had wished for.

The king grew hungry and weak, unable to eat or drink. Even his lovely daughter who rushed to his aid turned into a golden statue. Dismayed, the king realised that soon his whole kingdom would turn to gold unless he did something right away.

He begged the gods to turn everything back to the way it had been and to take back his golden touch. Because the king was ashamed and very sad, the kindly gods took pity on him and told him to go down to the river and bathe in its waters.

As Midas washed in the cold water he knew that not only had he lost his golden touch, but also his is desire for gold. So although he was poorer than he had been, he was richer, he felt, in the things that really matter.

☺ If you are still feeling sceptical about the law of attraction, start with something small. Often, people start by manifesting parking spaces. Once they are able to find perfect parking spots every time they need one, they are soon convinced.

My attraction steps

1. I decided what I wanted.

2. I ensured my goal was stated in the positive – I want to be healthy and physically fit.

3. I thought about it as though I had already achieved it.

4. I imagined how wonderful I felt and how amazing my life was now I had achieved it.

5. I kept that feeling.

6. I felt real gratitude for the things I already had and the things that were on the way to me. I did not just think blandly: I am grateful – I really felt it.

7. I repeated this step several times a day.

8. I accepted that my desire was already on its way.

9. I put any big, long-term goals on my vision board.

Putting a Goal into Your Future

Although many people are not aware of it consciously, we all have our own personal timeline. There are many techniques based around using a timeline to overcome past events, change limiting beliefs and release negative emotions. It is also very effective at increasing one's ability to achieve goals.

It is almost like putting the goal in the diary of your unconscious mind, so that you can unconsciously take the necessary decisions to achieve your goal.

Try the following:

1. Think about your life – your past and your future – as a line outside your body; even though you might not realise it, we all store time in this way. There is no right or wrong way for the line to run – however it is for you is perfect. Some people find that their timeline runs through them, whereas for others it does not touch the body.

2. Think intently about your goal.

3. Make it into a movie.

4. Make the sounds louder, the colours brighter, until it is really appealing.

5. Remember a pleasant event from your past.

6. Notice where that event would be on your timeline.

7. Think about a pleasant, planned event in the future like a holiday or Christmas.

8. Notice where it is on your timeline.

9. Now you have established where your past and future are.

10. Imagine yourself floating all the way out into your future above your timeline, carrying your goal with you.

11. Stop when you reach the place on the line where you believe is the date you have set for achieving your goal.

12. Take a deep breath and as you breathe out, energise good thoughts into your goal.

13. Think about how you will feel when you have achieved it or imagine telling those you care about of your achievement.

14. Repeat steps 12 and 13 three times.

15. Gently let go of your goal and allow it to float down into your timeline.

16. Float back to now and become aware of your present surroundings.

My golden goal grabber

I love achieving goals, so I developed the process of achieving the things I want into a simple, step-by-step process that has never failed me. I am so accustomed to achieving the things I desire that I honestly feel like the outcome is a certainty as soon as I have decided on my goal.

Start by using this process on some simple goals and then, as you begin achieving them with ease, you will find yourself moving on to bigger things with confidence:

1.   Decide what the main point of your goal is.

2.   Give it a timescale.

3.   Decide what your measures of success will be.

4.   Add all the other aspects of your life to the goal; give it real detail.

5.   Commit it in writing.

6.   Read it every day for the next week, just to see if anything comes up, like things that you have missed that you want to add or things that don't feel quite right.

7.   Then, when you are completely happy with it, show it to someone in your family to check if it fits in with their goals – like your spouse or partner, for instance.

8.   Make a vision board and look at it once a day.

9.   Decide what your smaller goals will be along the way.

10. Put it into your future on your timeline.

11. Use the law of attraction to guide your actions, act on your instincts and make your goal happen.

12. Take at least one action, no matter how small, every day to move you towards your goal.

☺ Step 7 is not essential for everyone but for me my husband is such a fundamental part of my overall happiness that I like to do this extra check, to confirm that we are aiming in the same direction.

Accepting Responsibility

Some people find the law of attraction hard to accept simply because it states that they are responsible for attracting to them everything in their lives, both good and bad. Others like to use the law or attraction as another scapegoat – I did not get what I want so it doesn't work.

So please let me reassure you that accepting responsibility for where you are and your results is not about blaming yourself for what you have attracted to you. If I blamed myself for bringing all the illnesses I have had upon myself, I would feel pretty bad. But I do believe I was responsible for them. Responsibility is not blame.

Years ago, when I attracted all my illnesses to me, I did not know anything about the power of the mind or the mind–body connection. As you will remember from my story, my tumours were discovered almost immediately after I set my goal of living until I am ninety-seven and finding them certainly saved my life.

> ☺ Obviously I have no way of knowing right now if I will achieve my goal, but my belief that I will has meant that the years since my illness have been incredibly happy. Plus, I do not fear going to the hospital for my scans and neither do I spend my life worrying.

Blame culture

Our society appears to foster the attitude that if something does not meet our expectations then we should assume it is someone else's fault. We can see this attitude in action all around us, in the people we know. They are easy to spot by the things they say: if the house is mess then nobody else is doing their fair share; if something is missing then someone else has moved it; if their income does not stretch to the end of the month either their spouse is wasting money or the company is not paying them enough.

Often, very early on in our sessions my clients tell me who is to blame for their problems. Sometimes they will be extremely hard on themselves, talking about themselves in such a harsh and nasty way that if someone else spoke about them like that, they would be incredibly hurt. More often, though, they will tell me about other people who are responsible for their lack of happiness, wealth or health. Usually it is a parent, spouse or even their own children.

It is gratifying to accept that you are responsible for where your life is going to be in twelve months' time. So I am asking you to rid yourself of any tendency to blame others or your past for where you are right now. Realise that you have choices and that even not making the decision to make changes in your life is still making a choice to stay just as you are.

Summary

If you have ever noticed a fly trapped in a room, although it is desperately seeking a way out and it is highly motivated, it keeps banging against the window.

> ☺ I will be honest – this drives me insane and I always open the window to let it out.

Unfortunately, many people exhibit similar behaviour. Despite lots of determination, they keep doing things that are ineffective.

You may have heard the expression that if something doesn't work then try and try again. Well, I firmly believe that if something isn't working, you should adapt your behaviour. The results you have in your life right now are the result of past behaviour. If you are thrilled with where your life is, that is fantastic. But if you think things could be better, look for ways of getting different results by changing your behaviour. Try something else.

Many fibromyalgia/CFS sufferers spend a great deal of money on pills and treatments in the hope of finding a cure, without ever changing their behaviour. My programme is based on looking inward for answers and changing your behaviours to get the results you want. So if you have had years of suffering and searching for a cure, resolve today to stop banging against the window – commit to my programme and take your path to recovery.

Key Steps to My Recovery

1. Set goals that are specific, measurable, congruent, achievable and time-bound.

2. Use the golden goal grabber.

3. Accept responsibility for your results.

4. Take action.

5. Create a vision board.

Chapter Twelve – The Secret of a Happy Life

> Each morning when I open my eyes I say to myself:
> I, not events, have the power to make me happy or
> unhappy today. I can choose which it shall be.
> Yesterday is dead, tomorrow hasn't arrived yet. I
> have just one day, today, and I'm going to be happy
> in it.
>
> Groucho Marx

Choosing Happiness

We would all choose happiness – or would we? Often when I ask
my clients to choose happiness, they say things like:

- How can I be happy when my marriage is a mess?
- I'm ill – how can you expect me to be happy?
- Would you be happy if you were in pain?
- I don't have enough money to be happy.

They are totally shocked when I tell them that happiness is not
dependant on what is happening in their life or on what they have or
don't have in material terms.

I believe true happiness comes from within. It comes from a person's perception of their situation, their current level of self-esteem and in meeting their emotional needs. Of course, there are events in life that make most people unhappy, like the death of a loved one. But what I am referring to is an individual's general underlying level of happiness on a daily basis.

The exercises throughout this book will greatly increase your feelings of happiness and contentment, if you use them effectively. But I want you to be able to achieve the life of your dreams, so this chapter is designed to help you understand what really makes you happy so you can change the way you feel at any given moment.

Learning to be happy

To a very large degree, the measure of our happiness is determined by how much we are able to live in the present moment. It is about appreciating what we have right now instead of focusing on what we don't have, without worrying about tomorrow, yesterday, last year or even what happened a decade ago.

Worrying about past problems and anticipated problems in the future is commonplace. Indeed, most people allow these thoughts to interfere with life on a daily basis. This means that the enjoyment they could be getting from the present moment is greatly reduced. In fact, the pleasure people feel can be reduced to the extent that they rarely experience real joy. This can lead to feelings of unhappiness, frustration and depression, which in turn can lead to sleepless nights and a worsening of fibromyalgia/CFS symptoms.

All too often people will postpone happiness, convincing themselves that some day they will be happy, some day things will get better. I will be happy when I've lost weight; I will be happy when I'm well; I'll be much happier when the children are at or have left school. There are several problems with this way of thinking:

1. People who think like this tend to find that when they reach their goal or obtain their desire, any happiness or elation they feel only lasts for a very brief time. This is because they immediately look to the next thing they feel they need in order to achieve happiness.

2. What they are doing is missing out on the happiness they could be feeling right now by postponing happiness. In essence, they are deleting all the good feelings they could be having by only focusing on what is wrong or on what could go wrong.

3. They are actually making it harder to achieve their goal, because we know from the teachings of the law of attraction that the fastest way to get what you want is to *feel* the emotion now that you are expecting it to bring. Put simply, if you believe a new car will make you happy, you need to learn to feel happy and appreciate what you have now.

No one has any guarantee that he or she will be here tomorrow. Now is the only moment that we have any control over. The past has gone and cannot be changed and we do not know for certain what will happen in the future.

Most people find it very difficult to be excited about their future yet they find it so easy to worry about it. I was certainly guilty of this and now I realise how destructive it was to think that way. Not only did I spoil my enjoyment of life, but I also spent so much time predicting what could go wrong that I actually brought those events into my life via the law of attraction. Then I justified my negative thoughts with the fact that I had been right.

Happy visualisation from the outside in

1. Smile – even though you might not feel like it right now, make it a really big smile.

2. Put on some happy music or sing a happy tune that you know well.

3. Sit up straight and hold your head up high.

4. Focus on your breathing.

5. Take a deep breath and hold it for a count of ten.

6. Release the breath slowly while counting to five.

7. Repeat the breathing exercise ten times.

8. Recall a happy memory while breathing normally and smiling.

9. Run the movie of the memory in your mind.

10. Imagine your happy memory as a small golden ball inside your head.

11. Allow it to spin slowly.

12. Visualise it gradually getting faster and spreading light.

13. Imagine the ball of happy light travelling throughout your body, spreading light with a tingling sensation of happiness.

Did you feel a change in the way you felt? If not, don't worry. Keep practising and you can become an expert at changing your mood, no matter what is happening in your life at the time.

Life is Not Fair

We can moan all day long about the injustices of life and we can rant about how some people are born with all the advantages, but the fact is it won't change a thing. We are not all born equal either physically or socially.

So accept the reality that life is not fair and instead of focusing on what you *don't* have, begin to focus on what you *can* do with what you have and where you are right now.

> ☺ I have no regrets about my background because it helped shape who I am today. And I can look back with fondness on amusing moments, like the time we had second-hand wallpaper! Honestly, it's true. It was taken down from our neighbour's fireplace wall in full lengths and put up on ours.

If you actually look for them, the world is filled with inspirational stories of people who have overcome amazing odds to achieve fantastic things. These are the type of people who should be the heroes and heroines of our society. Instead, we focus on reading magazines about the lives of the rich and famous, feeling jealous of their glamorous lifestyle, and then are secretly pleased when they fall off their pedestal. We compare ourselves to friends, family and neighbours who we perceive as having a better life than ours. But in reality we have no idea what is really going on in their lives. We cannot be certain that the happy veneer they display to the world is real. But if it is real then learn to be genuinely pleased for them – because this is the quickest way to attract happiness into your own life.

Ill Health Affects My Life, Can I Really be Happy?

Sadly, your aches and pains or lack of mobility may be with you for a long time. But that does not mean that your life cannot be amazing or that you cannot achieve great things and enjoy the world around you.

The Olympic Games are inspirational, but for me the Paralympics are far more so. Not only are these people great athletes, but they also overcame personal social and physical barriers to achieve their goals and dreams. I believe that being healthy is extremely important, but thankfully the world is filled with inspirational people who are able to inspire us not to let our physical inabilities hold us back.

Nick Vujicic was born in Melbourne, Australia, with the rare Tetra-amelia disorder: limbless, missing both arms at shoulder level and having one small foot with two toes protruding from his left thigh. Despite the absence of limbs he surfs, swims and plays golf and soccer. Nick graduated from college at the age of 21 with a double major in accounting and financial planning. He now travels around as a motivational speaker, focusing on helping teenagers.

We don't all have to go out and inspire others, win medals or compete in any field. But if we have personal goals, no matter how small they might appear to others, we are giving ourselves a sense of purpose and something to look forward to that we can celebrate.

Is There an Easier Way?

Are you one of those people who think that everything in life has to be a struggle? Do you dismiss the simple answers because you think they cannot possibly be the right ones? Often, the answers that come to us easily are delivered to us from our unconscious mind. Sometimes the simplest answer can be the right one, but learning to trust our instincts takes time. The following tips will build confidence in your own instincts.

Starting small is the first step towards trusting your instincts. For instance, you can decide how to spend your day. Should you try going out, pushing yourself to go shopping? Instead of going over all the possibilities and potential consequences in your mind, simply close your eyes and breathe deeply. Ask your mind: What is the best way for me to spend today? Trust the answer that instinctively pops into your head.

Tracking your progress is important. As you master the art of trusting your instincts when making small decisions, you will gradually become more confident using the technique for bigger and more important ones as well. Whenever you face a problem, avoid trying to over-think every possible option or aspect. Keep a note of the number of decisions which have turned out well and how often you feel another decision would have been better.

Most people stop trying to master this technique the first time their instinct appears to have been wrong. But it takes time to tune in to our instincts, so try again and persevere.

There is Always an Easier Way

> Legend has it that Gordious, Midas' father and the King of the Phrygia, learned of a special wagon that was situated in the Temple of Zeus. The pole of the wagon was tied to the wagon body using an intricate knot and the king decreed that whoever could unfasten the knot would go on to rule over Asia. Many tried to solve the puzzle and untie the knot, but none succeeded.
>
> Seized by a longing to test the prophecy, Alexander also tried to unfasten the knot by unravelling it, but when he was unable to do so, he drew his sword and cut right through it.

212

Even though he had not untied the knot in the way the king had expected, the king felt he had done what had been asked of him by getting to the heart of the matter and so he made Alexander the Ruler of Asia.

The Present Moment

The present moment is a gift, which many of us fail to appreciate. Actually being present in the moment can be difficult to achieve, particularly in the midst of the chaos of everyday life. The benefits of living in the present moment can be great, including:

1. Living life with a calmer, more relaxed awareness.

2. Greater enjoyment and appreciation of your daily life.

3. Overcoming the limitations you place on yourself.

4. Allowing yourself to be less affected by the negative actions of others.

5. Living your life intentionally rather than surviving it.

6. Being less negative.

It can be difficult to get your head around the realisation that only this one present moment exists. It is not a denial of yesterday, or your thoughts, experiences and memories, or the past. Neither does it mean ignoring the long- or short-term future. It is simply about accepting that when yesterday or last year were happening, it was the present moment and when tomorrow arrives, it will also be the present moment.

Animals always live in the present moment. They are completely immersed in what they are doing at any given moment. But thoughts will always wander – it is what minds do – and that is fine, as long as you can bring your attention back to the here and now at will. You operate more effectively and will get more enjoyment from everything you do by living in the present. If you have ever noticed a bird of prey flying through the trees turning and swooping on its prey, you will be witnessing the 100 per cent focus it demonstrates. Most first-class athletes have perfected this present-moment living, often referred to as being in the zone (see earlier).

We spend so much of our time being preoccupied with the past or the future that we are rarely completely alive. We miss the present moment, often reducing our enjoyment or experience. To be fully alive and experiencing life 100 per cent, we need to be fully in the moment. Now, this very second, is the only time that counts – it is all we really have. Only now are we truly alive. The past is gone, over, finished. The future has yet to happen – it isn't here yet. Thoughts about the future are not real. They are merely projections that take our focus away from the here and now. Living in the past and the future, and the absence of conscious living and being aware of the moment, is the cause of increased stress in many people's lives.

Simple ways to be in the moment

The next time you are walking down the street and it is safe to do so, fully focus on your experience. Switch off your iPod or put your mobile away for a few minutes. Become aware of the sounds you can hear around you. What can you see? Notice how your body feels as you move it. Are your arms swinging in a relaxed manner by your sides or are you holding yourself tense? Next, change the speed at which you are walking, first slowing down and then speeding up slightly. Notice the differences in how your body feels. Then walk normally again. Bring your attention fully back to your surroundings. Take in as much as you can. Don't analyse it, just enjoy the experience. You will be amazed how many things you have missed in the past.

When talking to your loved ones, listen with your full attention. Don't anticipate what they are going to say. Don't plan what you will say next. Instead, focus on their words, the tonality, the speed of their voice. Notice their body language. Be fully aware – see if they notice being really listened to.

If you are carrying out a routine task, one that you don't have to think about, your unconscious mind has taken it over for you, like brushing your teeth, having a shower or vacuuming. Actively engage in the task at hand and be completely present, just for a few minutes. Feel the sensations, notice any sounds, be aware of what you can see.

Schedule three times every day to stop and bring your attention inward. It can be done while waiting in a queue, when in a meeting or at any point when you are in danger of becoming lost in thought or your stress levels are rising. However, it is best to select three set times to do this practice until you are proficient at it.

To do this effectively you need to:

1. Acknowledge where your thoughts are at that moment.

2. Bring your attention in and focus on your breathing for twenty breaths.

3. Allow your awareness to expand to your entire body.

4. Notice any sensations you are feeling as you continue to breathe normally.

5. As you sense the life in throughout your body, you may detect a 'buzz' or a feeling of 'life' inside you.

It is fantastic to come back to the present moment and it is available to you at any time.

Living life in the present does not mean that you cannot reminisce about pleasant times or plan for the future. In fact, if you are living in the present moment, you are in the best place to plan for the future. This is because you will be relaxed and therefore have a clear mind to make good decisions.

Meditation – Step Four (Mindfulness Meditation: Thirty-minute Practise)

Mindfulness meditation is unique in that it helps us become present and aware of what 'is' at any given moment. It means accepting what is happening, no matter what it is, without trying to run from it or fight it.

People suffering from stress tend to spend the majority of their time focused on the past or the future. Mindfulness meditation is the practice of staying in the moment. This may appear to be a strange concept. After all, feeling stressed is often accompanied by feelings of wanting to escape from the reality of the current situation. People expend vast amounts of energy trying to run away and hide from, or fight, the discomfort or pain they feel as an inevitable part of living.

The surprising thing about mindfulness is that by immersing more deeply into the present moment, and into yourself just as you are already, and by accepting the moment as it is, it can bring about a sense of relaxation and calmness. The Buddha taught that we cause additional suffering by attempting to escape from our unpleasant experiences and by trying to prolong our pleasurable experiences. Instead of making us happier, this strategy has the opposite effect.

The concept of mindfulness is paying non-judgmental attention to the details of your experience as it arises and subsides. Instead of struggling to get away from experiences you find difficult, simply practise being with them. You might think that being present during pleasurable experiences is easy but, surprisingly, people spoil the experience by worrying that it won't last or by trying to keep it from fading away.

There are four aspects to this meditation technique that will enable you to focus on being present in the moment: body, breath, sounds and thoughts:

1. Sit either on a cushion on the floor or on a chair. If you choose a cushion you can use one that is designed for meditation practice like a zafu. Alternatively, you can use a meditation stool, a folded blanket or cushions.

2. If you choose to sit on a chair, your feet should be flat on the floor. If your feet don't reach the floor, you might need to put something on the floor for your feet to rest on. Adopt a posture that is upright and dignified.

3. If you choose to sit on the floor, simply cross your legs, ensuring you feel comfortable. Your hips should be higher than your knees. If necessary, sit on cushions or a folded blanket.

4. Rest your hands on your thighs, palms facing up.

5. Either close your eyes or soft focus your gaze on the floor in front of you about a metre away.

6. Begin by sitting in this position for a few minutes.

7. Next, bring your attention to your breath.

8. Notice it as it comes into your body and as it goes out.

9. Don't try to change the breath – simply notice it. Allow it to be however it is.

10. Continue to sit for a few minutes concentrating on your breath.

11. If your attention wanders, gently bring it back to your body and your breath.

12. Accept that your mind will wander; it is what minds do.

13. Whenever you notice that your mind has wandered, escort it back to the body and breath again.

14. Next, become aware of any sensations in your body. Just notice them. Perhaps you will notice warmth in one part; maybe even discomfort.

15. Simply notice the sensations and then come up close, paying attention to them with curiosity. Do not try to change anything; perhaps imagine breathing into the discomfort.

16. Bring your attention to any sounds. Notice the sounds in the room or perhaps outside. Don't label them – simply notice them.

17. Continue in this way for a few minutes.

18. Whenever you notice that your mind has wandered, escort it back to any sounds.

19. Finally, in this part of the practice, notice your thoughts. As you notice that thoughts arise, notice them being curious about them.

20. Imagine your mind is like the sky and your thoughts are birds. Notice if your thoughts are like a large flock of birds appearing all at once, swiftly crossing the sky as if in a rush to reach a far-off destination. Maybe single thoughts soar into view and quickly disappear again. Or do the thoughts linger like a bird of prey circling overhead?

21. When you realise that your attention has been focused on your thoughts, bring your attention back to the breath.

22. Finally, spend five minutes just being present in the moment. Notice your breath, any sensations in your body, any sounds or thoughts.

Do You Really Want to Recover?

This might sound like a strange question and I guess just the fact that you are reading this book means that you do want to recover. So it might surprise you to discover that not all sufferers will want to recover.

This does not make them crazy or bad in any way – it is simply that fibromyalgia/CFS has become such a big, important part of their life that it is now meeting one or more of their emotional needs. For example, joining a fibromyalgia/CFS support group may bring important friendships into an otherwise lonely existence, thereby meeting the need for connection; I will explain more later.

As you might find with overweight friends who appear to be undermining your healthy-eating regime, if you have any fellow sufferers who do not truly want to recover, beware that they might try to discourage you from focusing on your recovery, by preferring to discuss symptoms, etc. Be patient and understanding but firm and do not allow them to sabotage the good work you are doing.

Secondary gains

This is a psychiatric term meaning that a person has a hidden reason for holding on to an undesirable condition. In chronic pain management, where pain continues once an injury has healed, finding and releasing the perceived secondary gain can greatly contribute to healing. Examples of secondary gains include the attention one receives or monetary compensation for a disability.

Secondary gains are frequently unconscious, so I have no doubt that if I asked how much you want to recover, you would answer 100 per cent. But it is possible that deep in your unconscious mind there is a desire – that you are completely unaware of – to hold on to the condition.

Please don't dismiss this concept if you can't instantly think of anything, because as I explained, generally we are unaware of our secondary gains.

If you do not remove your secondary gain, what can happen is that you may put a great deal of energy into both practical and mind–body techniques to achieve your recovery but find it does not happen; in fact, it may even get worse. This is a signal that there may be an issue of secondary gain – that for some reason your unconscious mind feels more secure staying in your disadvantaged state rather than opting for improvement. In other words, your unconscious mind may be preventing your recovery because of a secondary gain that your unconscious mind believes to be of more importance than your recovery.

Removing your secondary gains

If you do find that you are not recovering as quickly as you might expect to, or indeed that you are getting worse, consider what your secondary gain could be. Once you have established that you have a secondary gain, look for practical ways to overcome it; this might involve discussions with those close to you.

It does not matter how small or insignificant the secondary gain may appear logically when compared with the terrible suffering of fibromyalgia/CFS – it may still be having an effect, so it is best to deal with it. If your recovery would mean returning to a job you dislike or having to do more household tasks you hate like ironing, either remove the perceived threat or change your perception of it.

It may surprise you to learn that I actually had a secondary gain, which if you think about it is obvious. As much as I hated being ill, it did have one advantage: I got to be a full-time mum. Okay, so it was not how I imagined it to be, but at least I was there for my daughter. I rid myself of my secondary gain by agreeing with my husband that no matter how well I became, my only job in life was to be happy and if that meant being at home then that is what I would do.

☺ I told you he is a saint! I am now working again, but doing something I love.

I have met some fibromyalgia/CFS sufferers who believe that if they recover without formal medical treatment, then it will prove to the sceptics that they were indeed faking or imagining the condition. I can understand these concerns as they certainly crossed my mind, but I realised that what mattered most was getting my life back and so I decided not to concern myself with what others might think.

Even if you don't feel you can tell anyone, be honest with yourself about your secondary gain; it might be vital to your recovery.

Stop talking about it

When you are not feeling well it is natural to want to talk about it – to tell people how you are feeling. This is particularly so when you have fibromyalgia/CFS, because you may look really well on the outside and so want to make them understand. If you have friends who are also suffering, it can seem comforting to share your experiences because let's face it – fibromyalgia/CFS is isolating. But the problem is that every time you talk about your symptoms, you are compounding and reinforcing them.

I now realise that I reinforced my symptoms by constantly telling myself – and my long-suffering husband if he was home – that I was in pain and exhausted. At the time he was wonderful about it and would do anything he could think of to ease my pain and make me feel better. But it was only after my recover that he admitted how bad and helpless it made him feel!

☺ Now, my husband enjoys listening to me chatter away happily. He says it is lovely to hear – like a babbling brook.

How I stopped talking about it

I made a conscious decision to stop talking about how ill I felt. From that day, if someone asked me how I was I answered: 'Great.' Even if I was having a bad day I would say: 'Good, thanks.' I was not lying, as there were many aspects of my life that were good. So even if my skin, neck or legs were hurting and I was feeling exhausted, I felt good about the fact that I was alive and that I could see the person and hear them asking me the question in the first place. I focused on what was right, rather than what was wrong in my life.

Once I stopped talking about me and instead asked them about their day or chatted for a few minutes about pleasant things, I felt better. This is because I had taken my focus off myself and the pain for a few minutes. In the beginning my focus would return to the pain or tiredness immediately, but gradually it took longer and longer, so I became a normal person rather than somebody who was just 'ill'.

For people who are going through a difficult time, support groups and forums can do an amazing job of preventing people from feeling isolated. But at the same time I recognised that the last thing I needed was to hear about other people's symptoms or problems they were experiencing. How can you possibly lean on someone who is already bent double? Think about it like this: if someone is telling you their legs are aching, the instant reaction from your unconscious mind is to become aware of your own legs to see if they are aching, too.

> ☺ With this in mind, I decided that the best way I could help other sufferers was to get better and then share how I did it. So I deliberately did not go on any forums or attend any support groups to learn more about my condition. And I have now written my book, which I hope will help you to begin your journey to recovery.

Dealing with Everyday Life

Whenever we are dealing with bad news, a difficult person or a disappointment of some kind, we can choose how to react to the situation. The problem is that many of us are in the bad habit of reacting negatively, which makes us feel worse. Most of us overreact, blow things out of proportion, focus on the negative aspects and hold on too tightly to the things we believe are important, even when we know deep down that we are wrong.

Many of my clients spend too much time thinking about what they don't have in their lives and hardly any time thinking about the good things they do have. Then they wonder why they feel sad, angry and fed up. Because they are feeling so low and negative, they get annoyed easily and become irrational and frustrated. For people with fibromyalgia/CFS, negative emotions drain our already limited energy and reduce our capacity for pain. As a result, because the pain and exhaustion increases, we feel more negative emotions, and everything spirals and seems worse; in other words, we lose sight of the bigger picture.

Making Problems Even Worse!

Some of us live life feeling like we are constantly going from one trauma to another, where everything seems like a big deal. If we continue to think like this, after a while we will end up believing that everything really is a trauma, telling ourselves it is because we are ill and cannot cope. What we fail to recognise is that the way we feel about problems has a lot to do with how quickly and efficiently we are able to resolve them, especially if we are manifesting them.

There is no doubt that some of you will have been through tragedies or will be facing real challenges right now or during your recovery from fibromyalgia/CFS and I will share with you how to deal with those situations later. But as you develop the habit of responding to life with more ease, problems that seemed insurmountable will begin to seem more manageable. Even the biggest of events will seem more within your control.

This is not to say that you can control everything that is happening in your life. What you have to do is ask yourself if there is anything you can do to improve this situation or deal with a particular problem. If the answer is yes, then take action and await the results. However, sometimes the answer will simply be no, there is nothing you can do to change the situation, in which case all you can do is choose how you react to it.

Not making things worse involves replacing old habits of obsessing and worrying, with new behaviours of accepting and dealing with problems without blowing them out of proportion. For example, if you are in the local supermarket and someone you know does not acknowledge your wave, do not automatically assume they have snubbed you or that you have done something to offend them.

Realise instead that they may be busy, distracted or even short-sighted and may not even have noticed you.

If you have burnt the dinner and have had to order a pizza, does this mean that you are a terrible wife, mother, husband or father, or does it just mean that tonight the family can have a treat? If I got upset every time I dropped a plate or smashed a glass while I was ill, I would have been constantly distressed. We just bought really cheap crockery that could be replaced easily.

One of the best things I ever heard for keeping things in perspective was to ask: Will it matter in six months? Quite honestly, for most of the situations we get stressed about the answer is no. If the answer is yes, it will still matter in six months, then I ask myself the following questions:

- What am I meant to learn from this challenge that will help me in the future?

- Who do I want to be in the face of this situation?

- What characteristics do I want to display that will enable me to handle this situation well?

- How can I handle this situation so that it gives me the best outcome?

I usually find the answers to these questions enable me to handle situations calmly and easily. If it is a situation where I need to let events happen at their own pace, I now feel able to do so. In the past, I would have tried to force a quick resolution because the uncertainly would have been overwhelming for me.

The Worst Thing That Could Happen

In ancient times in China there lived a very old man. Many thought he was over 120 years old and he was known to be very wise. Everyone in the nearby villages sought his advice and guidance. Then one summer's day, a farmer came to him in a state of panic.

'Wise sage, I don't know what to do. My ox has died and now I am unable to plough my fields. This is the worst thing that could ever have happened.'

The sage looked him in the eye and replied, 'Maybe so, maybe not.'

The farmer shook his head in disbelief, leaving without a word, certain this *was* the worst thing that could ever have happened.

The next morning the farmer went for a walk and in the distance he saw a strong young horse grazing in the field. Immediately, he had the idea to catch the horse and that his troubles would be over. He brought the horse back and realised how blessed he was, as ploughing was even easier than before.

As the people of the village congratulated him on his good fortune, the image of the sage came up in his mind and the man immediately went to visit the sage to thank him for his wise counsel.

Upon seeing the sage, the man said, 'Please accept my apologies. You were absolutely right. If I had not lost my ox, I wouldn't have gone on that walk and would never have captured the horse. You have to agree that catching this horse was the best thing that ever happened.'

The old sage looked into his eyes and said, 'Maybe so, maybe not.'

Surely this response must mean that the sage had lost his wisdom. Resolving not to visit the wise man again, the farmer returned home to the village.

Less than a week later the farmer's son was riding the horse back from the fields, when it was startled by group of children playing by the side of the road. Rearing up, it threw the farmer's son, breaking his leg. With his son unable to walk or work on the farm, the farmer was beside himself with panic. Again, the farmer went to the sage and told him what had happened.

'You are so wise; you saw the future and knew this would happen. Now, we will not be able to get all the work done; we will not have enough food. Surely now you must agree this is the worst thing that could ever have happened?' said the farmer.

Again the old sage, calmly and with kindness, looked into the farmer's eyes and replied, 'Maybe so, maybe not.'

The farmer was so furious with the response from the sage that he stormed off. Returning to his village, he informed his family that sadly, the sage had lost his mind and should not be consulted any more.

The very next day the emperor's army arrived and took all the young men to face almost certain death fighting in an impossible war. The farmer's son was the only young man not to be taken.

Meeting Your Own Needs

Anthony Robbins, Personal Development Guru, identified six basic emotional needs, which people are constantly and unconsciously trying to satisfy. In fact, all of our actions are aimed at meeting one or more of these needs, although we are often totally unaware of them:

1. Variety

In order to stop boredom, we need variety. Relationships become boring if everything stays the same. No matter how much people enjoy their job eventually, if there is no variety, they will become bored. How much variety or uncertainty people need depends on many personality factors, such as whether they are an extrovert or an introvert, for instance.

You may feel that you do not want or that you are unable to cope with variety or change. Perhaps you are not even be aware that lack of variety is an issue, if you have become very used to a set routine. If this is the case, remember a time when you did something different – perhaps a successful trip out or enjoying a different evening meal. As you remember the experience, consider how it made you feel better about your day. Next, make a list of ways you can build variety into your day in order for it to be more enjoyable.

I realise that this can be difficult with fibromyalgia/CFS, especially if your symptoms are severe – but it is not impossible, which is why I had so many hobbies. Even going to sit in the garden with a pair of binoculars and a book so you can identify the birds instead of being inside on the sofa adds some variety to your day. As you begin to recover, you can increase your variety in many other ways.

2. Certainty

In order to feel secure, we all need to know that some things are unlikely to change. But the world is constantly changing – the key is to develop the skills to handle any changes and challenges easily.

Many people will stay in an unhappy relationship or job they dislike because the fear of the unknown is even greater than the unhappiness they feel in the relationship or the position they currently find themselves in.

Some fibromyalgia/CFS sufferers may have felt relief when first given their diagnosis. This could be because they had received confirmation that their illness was not a terminal condition; however, they may also have felt relief because the element of uncertainty had gone.

The reason certainty is so important to us is because people fear they cannot cope if something bad happens. In the case of fibromyalgia sufferers, they often believe that they cannot face even nice changes, as everything becomes emotionally, as well as physically, overwhelming.

For me it was not just the feeling that I could not cope physically, it was that emotionally I was too tired to handle anything else. This was coupled with the belief that I was a failure because I had allowed myself to become ill with a condition that at the time I was not controlling.

3. Significance

We all need to know that we matter and that we are special in our own way. Often, we look to the outside world for our significance and are totally crushed when the people around us do not meet this need for us.

I am very lucky that my husband and daughter constantly do things to prove how significant I am to them. My career also increases my feelings of significance.

> ☺ But my real significance comes from inside me, because I know I am a good and worthwhile person – which is amazing when I consider how I used to feel.

I have had clients who have been highly successful and yet they felt like they were failing. This can happen when your internal filters are deleting, distorting and generalising the information around you in line with your belief that you are not good enough or when you put your significance on one particular aspect of yourself.

When I was suffering from fibromyalgia/CFS, I did not feel like I was being a good mother. Even though any energy I had went into caring for my daughter and stepchildren, I felt it was not enough. I wanted to be running around and playing with my daughter, not falling asleep on the sofa with my arms round her or hobbling down to the school with her. I wanted to prepare home-cooked meals, not pop something in the microwave.

But when I was diagnosed with my pancreatic tumour and had to face the fact that I might die, I was not worrying about who would walk her to school or cook her meals. I was terrified at the thought that I might not be there to listen to her tell me about her day. To listen to her problems and make her feel safe and loved. To tell her how incredibly proud she made me feel.

> ☺ I realised that day that throughout my seven years of fibromyalgia/CFS, I had still been a good mum because I had done all the really important stuff.

I know that for many people significance comes from possessions and wealth, and the respect they feel wealth can afford them. But this is only a very fragile significance, because all the wealth in the world will not make you feel really great about yourself. An actor client of mine recently shared how the adulation of fame had made him feel significant for a while and that as it faded, he was left with very low self-esteem. We see examples of this in the press every day, with celebrities constantly displaying more and more shocking behaviour or revealing personal details about their private lives in order to retain the attention.

4. Connection

Human beings are not suited to being solitary animals and we all need to feel a connection with or be loved by others to be truly happy. As we grow into adulthood, the need to achieve that connection outside the home becomes increasingly important. Forming appropriate and healthy relationships is vital to long-term happiness. To meet this need we can join a group or a club that has a positive purpose. While some may perform at extraordinary levels in order to be accepted, loved or connected as part of a high-achieving team, unfortunately, other people meet this need in a negative way by:

- joining gangs for a negative purpose
- becoming ill in order to feel connected and loved
- stealing
- taking drugs and drinking excessively to feel a part of a group and thereby achieve a sense of connection.

Everyone I know wants a life filled with love. But in order for this to happen, we must be a source of love rather than waiting for others to provide the love we need. We must *be* the people we want to attract and we must *give* the love, kindness and respect we want to receive. The best way that I know to bring more love into our lives is to look into our hearts and ask how we can *give* more love and *be* a greater source of love.

> ☺ If you want to feel more love in your life, put more emphasis on being a loving person and less on receiving love and you will have far more love in your life. It actually takes more energy to be negative and critical of others than it does to view them with an open and loving heart.

5. Contribution

The need to live a life that serves the greater good and the drive to go beyond ourselves is deep within us all. When we do this we experience true joy and fulfilment. A balance of contribution, to oneself and others, especially unselfish contribution, is the ultimate secret to the joy that so many people want in their lives.

6. Growth

Everything that is alive is either growing or dying. It doesn't matter how much money you have, how many people acknowledge you or what you have achieved in life – unless you feel like you are growing, you will be unhappy and unfulfilled. Growth is simply stretching yourself and doing more than you have achieved before. It is about learning and developing.

Achieving growth by expanding your comfort zone

We all live our lives within our comfort zones. It feels like a safe place, so why would we want to leave? Many of us live our lives like we have forever, but that is simply not the case. No matter how hard we resist, we will be forced at some point to leave our comfort zone because no one is protected from life's many challenges. It can be traumatic and stressful to be dragged out of our comfort zone to deal with a problem and people who are used to expanding their comfort zone deal with any issues with far more ease.

The good news is that every time you move outside your comfort zone, the new area you find yourself in becomes your new comfort zone. This means that you will feel comfortable and happy more of the time, even when faced with situations that might in the past have made you anxious. Growth is perhaps the most unidentified need, as people protest that they just want a peaceful, easy life.

> ☺ Unless you are completely happy and contented (in which case ignore my ramblings), I want you to decide to expand your world and live a truly interesting and exciting life.

The way to increase your comfort zone is very simple:

1. Do one thing every day that makes you feel slightly uncomfortable.

2. Acknowledge and celebrate your achievements, even if it is only in a small way.

3. Make bold, positive images of yourself in your mind.

4. Talk to yourself in a confident way.

5. Create positive, confident affirmations and repeat them often.

6. Think about someone who cares for or respects you. How do they see you? Which of your qualities do they admire?

> ☺ A simple thing to remember about all emotional needs is that if you give consistently that which you wish to receive, you tend to get it back from others.

Look at each of the emotional needs we have just covered and ask:

- How I am meeting this need currently?

- Is the way I meet this need good for me?

- Is the way I am currently meeting this need good for others around me and society as a whole?

- How can I improve the way I meet this need in the future?

Then simply plan how you can make changes to ensure all your needs are met in a way that is good for you, those close to you and society in general.

☺ You may find that the actions you take meet more than one of your needs at a time and maybe even all of them.

Look for the Extraordinary

Whatever you look for in life you will find it. If you want to find fault with your career, spouse, children, friend, relative or the world in general, you will certainly be able to do so. But if you choose to see the wonderful things in life you will find that they are all around you, too. When was the last time you really appreciated the beauty of nature, the smile of a child, the wag of your dog's tail when it greeted you?

☺ Honestly, I could go on forever – but I know that by now you are ready to find your own amazing things.

Everything Passes

When you are having a great time, it is almost as though time is flying and when you are having a difficult time or perhaps sat in the doctors surgery waiting for test results, it is as though someone has actually frozen time.

A fantastic strategy that has made a big difference to my life is to remind myself that everything passes, no matter how good or bad it appears at the time. Everything has a beginning, a middle and an end – that is the way life is. Every thought, experience or emotion you have ever had in your life is finished and has been replaced by another. It is human nature to want the pleasures in life to last as long as possible and for the unpleasant or painful experiences to be over immediately.

Experiment with the concept that everything passes, one present moment followed by another. Keeping this awareness close to your heart is not easy, especially in the face of adversity, but it is usually very helpful.

Asking Great Questions

Success guru Tony Robbins says: 'The quality of your life depends on the quality of your questions'. If you think about it logically, it is obvious that this statement is correct. I have transformed my life by asking the right questions. Consider these questions:

- Why has this happened to me?
- What have I done to deserve this?

If this is the type of question you ask yourself, your unconscious mind will go off looking for the answers to these questions and will come back with answers that, in accordance with your beliefs, explain how you reached your current situation. It may also fuel your belief that you are the victim of circumstances outside of your control and it is very unlikely that the information is going to move you forward to where you wish to be.

However, now look at these next questions:

- How can I move on from this point to improve my life?
- What is there in this situation that will help me live a happier life or move forward towards my goal?
- How can I enjoy the process of getting what I desire?
- What am I willing to do to get the results I want?
- What positive learning can I take from this experience?
- What steps can I take to improve my situation?

These questions are the type that successful, happy, healthy high-achievers all over the world ask themselves every day, with amazing results. It is a great place to start the transformation of your own life. So get asking!

When the Waters Were Changed

> Once upon a time a great god called upon mankind with a warning that all the water in the world that had not been specially saved would disappear in two weeks, to be renewed with different water, which would drive men mad.
>
> Only one man heeded the warning. He collected water in every vessel he could find and took it up into the hills, where he stored it and waited for the water to change. As the god had warned, all the water disappeared, so the man remained in his cave drinking his preserved water.
>
> When he saw the waterfalls again beginning to flow, the man descended from his cave and again walked among the people. He found that they were thinking and speaking in an entirely different way from before; yet, they had no memory or recollection of what had happened. When he tried to talk to them, he realised that they thought *he* was the one who was mad and they showed hostility towards him rather than compassion or understanding.
>
> He was dismayed and went back to the hills. Finally, however, because he could no longer bear the isolation of living alone, behaving and thinking in a different way from everyone else, he drank the new water and became like the rest. He became known as the madman who had regained his sanity.

Summary

The quickest way to get what you want in life is to learn to be happy with where you are, what you have and who you are right now.

Focusing on the good things in life and noticing the extraordinary or wonderful, even if they only last a moment, is something people with a positive and happy disposition do naturally. Thankfully, it is a skill we can all learn. That does not mean that you cannot desire or strive for change. It is simply about appreciating and feeling genuine gratitude for the good things that you have in your life right now.

If you do find yourself focusing on what is wrong in your life, either choose to stop and change the focus of your thinking, or ask the right questions to move your life in the right direction and change the way you feel. The more you focus on these aspects – instead of what is missing or wrong – the happier you will feel.

Key Steps to My Recovery

1. Practise being happy from the outside in.
2. Ensure you are meeting all the emotional needs.
3. Look for the wonderful in your life.
4. Ask great questions.
5. Feel happy now.
6. Accept that life is not fair or perfect.
7. Remove secondary gains.
8. Stop talking about it.
9. Realise that everything passes.
10. Stop making problems worse.

Final Note from the Author

Life is not measured by the number of breaths
we take, but by the moments that take our
breath away.

Author Unknown

You may have noticed that I have covered the four main problems
faced by fibromyalgia/CFS sufferers and that I have given you
techniques to help you overcome all of them. However, much of the
information given within these pages will help relieve more than one
symptom. For example, addressing your anxiety will reduce the pain
you feel and will give you more energy. Meditation and hypnosis will
help reduce all of your symptoms.

I have also introduced chapters covering the factors that I believe
are fundamental to a happy, healthy life. By following the techniques
in these chapters you will greatly accelerate your recovery and
improve every area of your life.

You may have been surprised how much of this guide to managing
fibromyalgia/CFS focuses on emotional and behavioural factors,
and that many of the techniques I have shared with you help you
deal with stress and other negative emotions. This is because I

believe that in most cases fibromyalgia/CFS is caused by secondary factors. By dealing with these you will get the double benefit of gaining better health, in addition to improvements in every area of your life.

I am sure you will be wondering how long it will take for you to recover, but I am afraid I cannot answer that for you. What I am sure of, however, is that the more diligently you apply my processes, the quicker it will be.

For me, the journey may have taken slightly longer than it will for you because I did not have a book like this one, in which someone was telling me the steps I had to take in order to recover. On the contrary, I had to go out, learn the techniques and adapt them for recovery from fibromyalgia/CFS. I suggest you do not put the pressure of a time limit on yourself, but if you want a timescale to aim for you should give yourself a period of at least six months before seeing any significant improvement.

I noticed almost immediately that I was feeling happier and more positive when adopting the techniques I have shared with you in this book. So despite not feeling well every day while I was recovering, I could still be cheerful, optimistic and enjoy life. Furthermore, as I explained in my story, this was even more amazing because at the time I was living through what most people would regard as a profoundly stressful period as a result of house renovations, financial difficulties and my other illnesses. These positive feelings have stayed with me and increased, so that most of the time I am genuinely blissfully happy.

> ☺ I am only human, however, and I do get lows like everyone else – they are just not as low as they used to be.

My Recovery in Brief

For me, the first thing that happened was that the bad days became fewer and farther between and the flare-ups did not last as long. My energy levels increased gradually as I got stronger and exercised more, and my tender points reduced in sensitivity until they disappeared altogether.

Within twelve weeks I was feeling great almost every day. The only time I felt exhausted was just before my menstrual period. Nothing improved in this sense for about six months, but gradually this reduced to the normal drop in energy levels that many women experience during this time. Interestingly, the last tender point to disappear was my left shoulder blade and the last area in which I felt pain was in my left thigh.

It was approximately six months into my recovery that the growths in my kidney, and then the pancreas, were discovered and then of course I had the operation and MRSA to contend with – and shortly after that the malignant melanoma. But despite all the pressures of life-threatening illnesses, operations and financial concerns when my husband had to resign from his job to care for me and our daughter after my operation, my resolve to recover increased and I remained determined to recover and enjoy my life. If I had a bad day I focused on the fact that it would pass and recognised that without my techniques, there probably would have been far more bad days to contend with.

This marks the end of the book but possibly the beginning of your journey to better health and a fantastic life. I hope my journey has inspired you and given you hope that you, too, can recover. Please remember these four things as they will help you manage your fibromyalgia/CFS:

- your unconscious mind is incredibly powerful
- you have the key within you to unlock its power
- many things have been thought impossible until someone did it, and
- life is a journey, so begin with deciding on your destination.

    ☺ Remember: I am just an ordinary person like you. I believe you can recover – do you?

Until we meet.

Rebecca Richmond

If you wish to continue your journey with my help, please visit my website to find out about the ways you can continue to work with me through my CD recovery programme with pre-recorded meditations and hypnosis:

<http://www.forgetfibomyalgia.com>

Index

134, 146, 151, 160, 189, 226

forgiveness 126, 129, **126–31**, 148, 152

frustration 4, 21, 40, 54, 55, 84, 90, 122, 123, 124, 162, 181, 208, 222

guilt 14, 21, 37, **126**

happiness . 32, 37, 55, 92, 116, 138, 139, 146, 149, 152, 191, 199, 228, 230, 232, **207–35**, 236

helplessness 40, 132

joy 43, 133, 161, 208, 209, 211, 213, 214

mood . 37, 78, 81, 85, 88, 112, 115, 123, 170, 210

negative ... 59, 65, 78, 98, 104, 122, 130, 137, 156, 181, 199, 201, 222, 228

nervousness.... 43, 126, 138

sadness................ 122, 222

stress 3, 16, 24, 46, 47, 52, 53, 56, 72, 80, 83, 84, 88, 91, 97, 101, 104, 122, 126, **131–35**, 161, 214, 215, 227, 229, 235

tension 104, 126

unhappiness 152, 187, 208, 226, 229

well-being . *See* self-esteem

worry ... 43, 52, 57, 84, 85, 104, 126, 131, 132, 133, **141–43**, 161, 208, 209, 216, 222

endorphins **101**, 102, 103, 115, 128

energy 47, 48, 51, 52, 54, 55, 56, 61, 62, 67, 72, 81, 82, 91, 92, 104, 106, 110, 128, 130, 131, 159, 160, 168, 173, 175, 177, 181, **183**, 199, 215, 219, 222, 235, 237

vampires **157, 158**

enjoyment......... *See* emotions

events 3, 6, 35, 36, 37, 38, 39, 40, 44, 53, **57–59**, 80, 100, 104, 123, 124, 126, 131, 135, 137, 146, 151, 161, 162, 187, 201, 202, 208, 209, 222, 223

exercise .. 15, 48, **65–70, 65–73**, 99, 101, 102, 113, 156

stretching 99

yoga 69

Glossary of Terms

Acupuncture: complementary medicine during which fine needles are inserted into the skin at specific points along what are considered to be lines of energy.

Acute: (of a disease or its symptoms) severe but of short duration.

Adenosine: a chemical messenger which plays an important role in biochemical processes, such as energy transfer. It is also an inhibitory neurotransmitter, believed to play a role in promoting sleep and suppressing arousal, with levels increasing with each hour a person is awake.

Adrenaline: hormone secreted by the adrenal glands that increases the body's rates of blood circulation, breathing and carbohydrate metabolism, and prepares muscles for exertion.

Affirmation: action or process of affirming something.

Alternative therapy: medical therapy not regarded as orthodox by the medical profession, such as crystal healing, naturopathy and herbalism.

Anchors: stimuli that call forth states of mind, which are thoughts or emotions, and then corresponding actions.

Angiomyolipoma: a rare, well-known soft tissue tumour that can achieve a large size and is usually benign.

Belief: an acceptance that something exists or is true, especially one without proof.

Benign: (of a disease) not harmful in effect. Not malignant (of a tumour).

Bioenergy: renewable energy produced by living organisms.

Biopsy: examination of tissue, removed from a living body in order to discover the presence, cause or extent of a disease.

Brainstem: the central trunk of the mammalian brain, consisting of the medulla oblongata, pons and midbrain.

Calories: unit used to measure the energy value of foods.

CFS: chronic fatigue syndrome. A medical condition of unknown cause with fever, aching, prolonged tiredness and depression, typically occurring after a viral infection.

Cholesterol: a waxy substance produced by the liver and found in certain foods, needed to make vitamin D and some hormones.

Chronic: (of an illness) persisting for a long time period or constantly recurring.

Circadian rhythm: any biological process that displays an oscillation of about twenty-four hours.

Circulation: continuous motion by which the blood travels through all parts of the body under the action of the heart.

Condition: an illness or other medical problem.

Conviction: a firmly held belief or opinion.

Coronary: relating to or denoting the arteries that surround and supply the heart.

Dehydration: loss of a large amount of water from the body.

Diabetes: a disorder of the metabolism causing excessive thirst and the production of large amounts of urine.

Dietician: an expert on diet and nutrition.

Diuretic: causing increased or excessive production and passing of urine.

Dopamine: a compound present in the body as a neurotransmitter and a precursor of other substances, including adrenaline.

EFT: form of counselling that draws on several areas of alternative therapy. Falls into the category of alternative medicine.

Endocrine system: collection of glands which secrete hormones that regulate metabolism, growth and development, tissue and sexual function, reproduction, sleep and mood, etc.

Endorphin: morphine-like painkilling substances that decrease pain sensation.

Endoscopic scan: an endoscope is an instrument that can be introduced into the body to give a view of its internal parts.

Energy meridians: invisible lines through the body that carry energy to every organ and system.

Fatigue: extreme tiredness often resulting from illness or mental or physical exertion.

Fibro (brain) fog: term used to describe lapses of memory or concentration in sufferers of fibromyalgia.

Fibromyalgia: a rheumatic condition characterised by muscular or musculoskeletal pain with stiffness and localised tenderness at specific points on the body.

Herpes: any of a group of virus diseases caused by herpes viruses, affecting the skin (often with blisters) or the nervous system.

Hormones: a person's sex hormones as held to influence behaviour or mood; substances produced to trigger, stimulate or regulate particular body functions into action.

Hydrogenated vegetable oil: widely used manufactured fat product.

Hypnosis: trance-like state characterised by extreme suggestibility, relaxation and heightened imagination.

Hypothalamus: a portion of the brain with a variety of functions. One of the most important of which is to link the nervous system to the endocrine system via the pituitary gland.

Imagery: use of visual images.

Immune system: the organs and processes of the body that provide resistance to infection and toxins. Organs include the thymus, bone marrow and lymph nodes.

Inflammation: localised physical condition in which part of the body is reddened, swollen, hot and often painful, especially as a reaction to injury or infection.

Inner voice: internal monologue, internal speech or verbal conscious thinking in words. Internal dialogue is a conversation one has with oneself at a conscious or semi-conscious level.

Insoluble: (of a substance) incapable of being dissolved.

Intuition: the ability to understand something instinctively, without the need for conscious reasoning.

Irritable bowel syndrome: a widespread condition involving recurrent abdominal pain and diarrhoea or constipation, often associated with stress, depression, anxiety or previous intestinal infection.

Law of attraction: a belief or theory that like attracts like and that by focusing on positive or negative thoughts, one can bring about positive or negative results.

Ligaments: short bands of tough, flexible, fibrous connective tissue that connects two bones or cartilages or holds together a joint.

Lymph nodes: small glands of the immune system.

Malignant: virulent or infectious, tending to invade normal tissue or to recur after removal; cancerous.

Malignant melanoma: a rare and very serious type of skin cancer.

Mantra: word or sound repeated to aid concentration in meditation.

ME: the common name for myalgic encephalopathy, sometimes also known as Myalgic Encephalomyelitis. Can be severe and debilitating with fatigue, painful muscles and joints, disordered sleep, gastric disturbances, and poor memory and concentration.

Meditation: generally an inwardly oriented personal practice which individuals do by themselves, to achieve a deep sense of inner calm.

Menstrual period: a flow of blood and other material from the lining of the uterus (womb), lasting for a few days and occurring in sexually mature women who are not pregnant at intervals of about one lunar month until the menopause.

Metabolism: chemical processes that occur within a living organism in order to maintain life.

Methicillin-resistant Staphylococcus Aureus (MRSA): skin bacterium responsible for several difficult-to-treat infections in humans, that is resistant to a range of antibiotics.

Mind–body connection: where the mind and body work together to foster the healing process on a physical level.

Monounsaturated: saturated except for one multiple bond.

Motor skills: a learned sequence of movements that combine to produce a smooth, efficient action in order to master a particular task.

Nervous system: the network of nerve cells and fibres that transmit nerve impulses between parts of the body.

Neuron: an electrically excitable cell that processes and transmits information by electrical and chemical signalling.

Neurotransmitters: chemicals which, when released, activate other nerve cells in the spinal cord, to process the information and then transmit it up to the brain.

Non-REM sleep: stages of sleep that do not involve dreaming.

Nutrient: a substance that provides nourishment essential for the maintenance of life and for growth.

Omega-3 fatty acid: an unsaturated fatty acid of a kind occurring chiefly in fish oils, with double bonds between the carbon atoms that are third and second from the end of the hydrocarbon chain.

Osteoporosis: a medical condition in which the bones become brittle and fragile from loss of tissue, typically as a result of hormonal changes, or a deficiency of calcium or vitamin D.

Pancreas: a large gland behind the stomach that secretes digestive enzymes into the duodenum (first part of the small intestine).

Pancreatectomy: a major surgical procedure to remove all or part of the pancreas.

Pedometer: instrument for estimating the distance travelled on foot by recording the number of steps taken.

Physiotherapy: treatment of disease, injury or deformity by physical methods such as massage, heat treatment and exercise rather than by drugs or surgery.

Polyphenois: type of antioxidant.

Posture: a particular position of the body; the characteristic way in which someone holds their body when standing or sitting.

Rapid eye movement sleep (REM sleep): a normal stage of sleep characterised by the rapid and random movement of the eyes.

Reticular activating system (RAS): information-filtering system of the brain that evaluates incoming data.

Saturated: denoting fats containing a high proportion of fatty acid molecules without double bonds, considered to be less healthy in the diet than unsaturated fats.

Secondary gain: an often unconscious reason for a patient to hold on to an unwanted condition.

Selenium: chemical eliminate of which trace amounts are necessary for cellular function in many organisms, including all animals.

Sensory perception: stimuli a person processes and understands through their five senses: smell, sight, taste, touch and hearing.

Serotonin: a compound present in blood platelets and serum, which constricts the blood vessels and acts as a neurotransmitter; known as the 'feel-good factor'.

Sleep switch: designed to occupy the mind so it is impossible to focus on negative thoughts and to provide a powerful anchor for sleep.

Soluble: (of a substance) able to be dissolved, especially in water.

Sub-modality: any component that makes up a visualisation or an image; for example, whether it is black-and-white or colour.

Symptom: a physical or mental feature that is regarded as indicating a condition of disease, particularly such a feature that is apparent to the patient.

Synapse: a structure that permits a neuron to pass an electrical or chemical signal to another cell.

Syndrome: a group of symptoms which consistently occur together or a condition characterised by a set of associated symptoms.

Tapping: a simple but effective technique used for dealing with emotions and pain, in line with acupuncture pressure points.

Tender points: specific places on the body (eighteen specific points at nine bilateral locations) that are exceptionally sensitive to touch in people with fibromyalgia.

TFT: psychological treatment intended to heal a large variety of mental and physical ailments through specialised 'tapping' with the fingers at meridian points of the upper body and hands.

Time Line Therapy™: intervention developed by Dr Tad James and used successfully in conjunction with all NLP techniques.

Trans-fat: an unsaturated fatty acid with a trans arrangement of the carbon atoms adjacent to its double bonds.

Tumour: abnormal growth of tissue, whether benign or malignant.

Ulcer: open sore on external or internal surface of the body, caused by a break in the skin or mucous membrane which fails to heal.

Ultrasound scan: sound or other vibrations having an ultrasonic frequency, particularly used in medical imaging to examine the body.

Unconscious mind: part of the mind that is inaccessible to the conscious mind but which affects behaviour and emotions.

Vegan: person who does not eat or use animal products.

Vegetarian: a person who does not eat meat or fish, and sometimes other animal products, especially for moral, religious or health reasons.

Vision board: a simple yet powerful visualisation tool.

Visualisation: when someone forms a mental picture of something.

Whipple procedure: major surgical operation involving the pancreas and other organs. This operation is performed to treat cancerous tumours on the head of the pancreas.

Zone, the: when you are in 'the zone', you are in a state of relaxation, from which things come about effortlessly and easily.

About the Author

Author of several self-help books, Rebecca Richmond has enjoyed a highly successful career within global organisations, later going on to become a qualified coach. Having triumphed over adversity, fibromyalgia/CFS and cancer, as a coach and master practitioner of NLP, hypnosis and Time Line Therapy™, she is ideally equipped to help you achieve the wellness you deserve.

Other Books in the Series

My Guide: How to Write a Novel

My Guide: Overcome Insomnia

My Guide: Manage Chronic Pain

Coming Soon:

My Guide: How to Market & Sell Your Book

My Guide: Manage Stress Levels

My Guide: Increase Self-Esteem

My Guide: How to Write a Non-Fiction Book.

Health is a state of complete physical, mental and social well-being, and not merely the absence of disease or infirmity.

World Health Organization, 1948

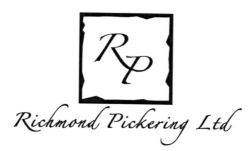

Richmond Pickering Ltd